I0448952

The Tender Road

Guiding Your Loved One Through Dementia

by
Joel F. Boyd

Copyright 2024 Joel F. Boyd. All rights reserved.

No part of this book may be reproduced in any form or by any electronic or mechanical means including information storage and retrieval systems, without permission in writing from the author. The only exception is by a reviewer, who may quote short excerpts in a review.

Although the author and publisher have made every effort to ensure that the information in this book was correct at press time, the author and publisher do not assume and hereby disclaim any liability to any party for any loss, damage, or disruption caused by errors or omissions, whether such errors or omissions result from negligence, accident, or any other cause.

This publication is designed to provide accurate and authoritative information with regard to the subject matter covered. It is sold with the understanding that the publisher is not engaged in rendering professional services. If legal advice or other expert assistance is required, the services of a competent professional should be sought.

The fact that an organization or website is referred to in this work as a citation and/or a potential source of further information does not mean that the author or the publisher endorses the information the organization or website may provide or recommendations it may make.

Please remember that Internet websites listed in this work may have changed or disappeared between when this work was written and when it is read.

Table of Contents

Introduction:
Journey into the Heart of Dementia

Embarking on the journey of caring for someone with dementia is akin to navigating a landscape shrouded in mist, where each step uncovers new challenges and poignant revelations. Through the fog of uncertainty, caregivers persist with a courage that often goes unseen, treading a path marked by emotional nuance and the imperative of adaptability.

Dementia, a term that encapsulates a myriad of cognitive disorders, stands as a testament to the fragility of the human mind. It whispers of times both gentle and unforgiving, where memories fray at the edges, and familiar faces become uncharted landmarks. Yet, within this journey into the heart of dementia, there exists a profound intimacy and a testament to the strength of the human spirit.

As a caregiver, you're embarking on a voyage where each day may bring its measure of sorrow and grace. Understanding the intricacies of dementia is paramount, not only for providing compassionate care but also for preserving the delicacy of the human connection that endures through the turbulence of disease.

The task before us is not to delineate the clinical definitions of dementia or chart the symptoms, for those explorations await in later chapters. Here, we delve into the heartfelt reality of caregiving, acknowledging the depth of adversity you face while illuminating the potential for unexpected joy and resilience in the face of cognitive decline.

It's within the sacred space of care that we find life's intricate dance between dependence and dignity. We witness the gradual metamorphosis of roles and relations, where once guided hands now become the guide. The dynamics of caregiver and cared-for rewrite themselves in the quiet moments of daily life, shaping a shared experience rooted in compassion.

This journey is a mosaic of minute and monumental moments, each crafting the narrative of a shared human experience. As you walk this path, the whisper of a forgotten melody, the half-light of a smile, or the tender clasp of a hand might emerge as the day's quiet triumphs.

In this introduction, we reflect on the essence of our travels into the heart of dementia, holding space for the emotional contours of such an odyssey. Like an impressionist's painting, each encounter with our loved one is a dab of color, contributing to a larger portrait of what it means to give and receive care.

But let's not wander in abstraction. Your role as a caregiver is incredibly difficult—fraught with decisions that weigh heavily on both head and heart. It's a labor not just of necessity but of love. This text serves as a guide to buoy you through the storms and help find your bearings when you feel adrift in the complexities of caregiving.

Throughout these pages, we'll explore the practical aspects of daily care, creating routines, and crafting a safe environment, with the acute awareness that even the most meticulous planning must yield to the fluidity of your loved one's needs and capabilities. You'll encounter strategies and support to shore up your resilience and preserve the wellspring of your own well-being. For within the boundless demands of caregiving, neglecting one's own health and happiness serves neither caregiver nor recipient.

Your journey is a shared narrative with countless others who find themselves in this compassionate calling. We'll explore the power of connections, those formed within the sanctuary of support groups, or across the ether of online platforms. Here, you can forge bonds that serve as lifelines, offering solace and wisdom in equal measure.

As we begin, remember that this trek is not marked by the solitary figure of a caregiver standing vigil but by a community that embraces each step, each victory, each setback together. The path of dementia care is not just about loss or the slow ceding of faculties; it's equally about the moments of profound connection that defy the ravages of disease.

Embarking on this journey, we acknowledge the many facets of dementia care—not just the strains but also the strengths it can unveil within us. We celebrate not only the endurance of caregivers but their capacity to find grace in the midst of the gradual goodbyes.

With that spirit of profound respect and recognition, let us step forward, honoring the layers of this journey into the heart of dementia. For within the shadows cast by this condition, there can still be the warmth of moments illuminated by understanding, patience, and love. This is your guide, your companion on a path that speaks of life's delicate balance and the enduring nature of compassion and connection.

Chapter 1:
Understanding Dementia and Its Effects

Dementia is a pervasive condition that touches the lives of millions around the globe. It's a term that conjures both understanding and misunderstanding in equal measure. Broadly, it refers to a decline in cognitive function beyond what might be expected from normal ageing. But to truly comprehend its impact, we must delve deeper, examining not just the individual it touches but the ripple effects it has on families, caregivers, and communities.

At its core, dementia can arise from various causes with Alzheimer's disease being the most well-known and prevalent. Alzheimer's, like other forms of dementia, gradually diminishes a person's ability to process thought, affecting memory, understanding, judgment, language, and more. However, it's crucial to recognize that each type of dementia brings its own unique set of challenges and symptoms, painting a diverse picture of cognitive decline.

The typical symptoms associated with dementia profoundly alter not only cognitive functions but also behavior and daily functioning. Memory loss, confusion about time or place, difficulty handling money or making decisions, and changes in personality and behavior are hallmarks of the condition. These symptoms eventually lead to a significant shift in an individual's ability to perform everyday activities, creating a cascading effect on their independence and quality of life.

Witnessing the cognitive decline of a loved one is a deeply emotional journey, characterized by a rollercoaster of emotions ranging from denial and frustration to deep sorrow and empathy. The gradual loss of independence that comes with dementia is particularly challenging, as once-capable individuals find themselves increasingly reliant on others for their basic needs and daily activities.

This shift in independence often precipitates a change in the dynamics between caregivers and care recipients. Roles may reverse, and relationships can become strained as caregiving responsibilities increase. It's a transition that requires patience, understanding, and, most importantly, a compassionate acknowledgment of the new reality both parties are facing.

As we delve into the impacts of dementia, it becomes evident that the condition does more than just impair memory and cognitive function. It challenges the very essence of relationships, forcing us to adapt and grow in ways we might not have anticipated. The caregiver's role evolves from one of companion and family member to include responsibilities akin to those of healthcare professionals, albeit steeped in familial love and concern.

Understanding dementia requires more than just a familiarity with its clinical aspects; it necessitates a deep empathy for those it affects and an appreciation for the profound emotional journey undertaken by caregivers and families. The emotional impact of witnessing a loved one's cognitive decline can be overwhelming, leading to feelings of helplessness and despair.

However, amidst the challenges, there are moments of profound connection and joy to be found. Recognizing and embracing these moments can provide both the caregiver and the person living with dementia a sense of normalcy and happiness, even if fleeting.

Such recognition also brings to light the importance of navigating the changing dynamics in the caregiver and care recipient relationship with grace. Finding a balance between providing care and fostering independence where possible can help maintain the dignity of the person living with dementia.

The journey through dementia is one of gradual adjustment to a new normal, both for those directly experiencing its effects and for their loved ones. Understanding the nuances of the condition, including the emotional and psychological toll it takes, is the first step toward compassionate care.

Comprehending dementia's effects also involves acknowledging the unpredictability of the condition. Symptoms can fluctuate, presenting good days alongside more challenging ones, making flexibility and patience key components of effective caregiving.

In striving to understand dementia, we must also learn about the resources available to support both those living with the condition and their caregivers. From medical interventions to supportive communities and practical tips for daily care, knowledge is a powerful tool in managing the challenges that dementia presents.

Ultimately, understanding dementia and its effects is about creating a foundation of empathy and support that enriches the lives of everyone involved. It's about providing care that honors the individual, cherishes the moments of clarity and joy, and navigates the challenges with kindness and understanding.

In this journey, caregivers play a crucial role, not only in providing practical care but in maintaining the emotional and psychological well-being of their loved ones. Their resilience, love, and dedication are the bedrock upon which the daily realities of living with dementia are borne.

As we move forward, let's carry with us the understanding that dementia, while challenging, also presents opportunities for growth, compassion, and deeper human connection. Armed with knowledge and empathy, caregivers and families can navigate this journey with grace, finding moments of joy and fulfillment amidst the trials.

Defining Dementia and Its Causes

As we journey further into the exploration of dementia, it becomes crucial to understand what exactly this condition entails and the multiple factors that lead to its onset. Dementia is not a single disease but a collective term used to describe a range of symptoms associated with a decline in memory, reasoning, and other thinking skills. Various diseases can cause it, with Alzheimer's disease being the most common trigger. However, dementia can also stem from vascular issues, Parkinson's disease, Lewy body dementia, and frontotemporal dementia among others. These conditions lead to damaged nerve cells in the brain, affecting their ability to communicate, which in turn impacts the person's behavior, emotions, and physical functions. This breakdown in communication signifies the beginning of a challenging journey for both the individual and their caregivers, emphasizing the importance of understanding the underlying causes to provide the most effective care.

Overview of Alzheimer's Disease and Other Types of Dementia

In our journey to understand dementia, it's pivotal to grasp the nuances and variances among its types, most notably Alzheimer's disease, which unfurls its narratives in the hearts and minds of many affected. This exploration not only aims to enlighten but also to arm caregivers with the knowledge needed to navigate the complex challenges ahead.

Dementia, a term shrouding a multitude of cognitive impairments, affects millions globally, with Alzheimer's standing as its most infamous culprit. This condition insidiously strips away memory, thinking skills, and the very essence of one's personality, often likened to the slow dimming of a once brilliant light. Alzheimer's, however, is but one thread in the intricate tapestry of dementia varieties, each with distinct origins, symptoms, and trajectories.

While Alzheimer's disease accounts for an estimated 60 to 80 percent of cases, other types such as vascular dementia, Lewy body dementia, and frontotemporal dementia etch their marks profoundly. Vascular dementia, often emerging in the wake of a stroke, delineates a path of cognitive decline paralleled by physical ailments. Lewy body dementia, punctuated by its telltale deposits in brain cells, weaves a complex pattern of symptoms, including striking visual hallucinations and sleep disturbances.

Frontotemporal dementia, on the other hand, casts a shadow predominantly over personality and language, gradually eroding the ability to communicate and interact meaningfully with others. This rare form breaks the mold by frequently affecting individuals at a comparatively younger age, painting a starkly different portrait of dementia.

Understanding the diverging paths these illnesses take is crucial for caregivers tasked with navigating the unpredictable waters of dementia care. Each type mandates a unique approach, tailored strategies, and an immense reservoir of patience and empathy. Acknowledging these differences fosters a more nuanced comprehension of the challenges a caregiver and their loved one may face, allowing for a response that's both informed and compassionate.

The struggle with Alzheimer's and its cousins extends beyond memory lapses to encompass difficulties in planning, reasoning, and problem-solving, often leaving individuals feeling adrift in their familiar surroundings. Behavioral changes, too, emerge as daunting obstacles, with mood swings and withdrawals casting long shadows over daily life.

Moreover, it's imperative to highlight the importance of early detection and the role of medical intervention in managing symptoms, albeit there is no known cure for Alzheimer's and most other types of dementia. Therapeutic strategies and medications can, however, slow the progression and improve quality of life, making moments of clarity and connection all the more precious.

Additionally, the introduction of lifestyle modifications and supportive therapies opens avenues for engaging the affected individual in meaningful activities, thus harnessing remnants of memory and cognitive functions for as long as possible. Diet, exercise, and cognitive stimulation emerge not only as pillars of prevention but also as beacons of hope in the management of dementia's symptoms.

The evolution of dementia, including Alzheimer's disease, does not adhere to a singular narrative but rather unfolds in a multitude of ways, each influenced by a person's history, genetics, and environmental factors. This mosaic of influences underscores the complexity of providing care that addresses not only the medical but also the emotional and social needs of those affected.

Equally, the progression into later stages of dementia paints a somber picture, characterized by an increased dependence on caregivers. The transition from mild forgetfulness to profound impairment demands a continuum of care, compassion, and understanding, requiring caregivers to adapt constantly to evolving needs.

In sum, the tableau of Alzheimer's and other dementias is intricate and multifaceted. For caregivers stepping into the role of guardians, educators, and confidants, knowledge of these distinctions is a beacon in the fog of uncertainty. It's a journey fraught with challenges yet marked by moments of profound connection and deeply human experiences.

As we delve further into the specifics of care strategies and support mechanisms in subsequent chapters, let us carry forward this foundational understanding of the varied landscape of dementia. It is with this knowledge that we can approach caregiving with the insight, empathy, and resilience required to make a meaningful difference in the lives of those walking the tender road of dementia.

Indeed, the path of a caregiver is not linear but winding, marked by trials and triumphs alike. Bearing the weight of this responsibility with grace and fortitude requires not just love but an understanding of the dragon you face. Alzheimer's disease and its brethren in dementia represent formidable foes, yet armed with knowledge and a compassionate heart, caregivers can and do rise to meet them head-on.

The journey through dementia is a testament to the strength of the human spirit, both in those who navigate its troubled waters and in those who stand steadfastly by their side. In understanding Alzheimer's disease and other types of dementia, we find not only the tools to fight back but also the wisdom to appreciate the moments of joy, of clarity, that shine all the brighter against the backdrop of adversity.

Typical Symptoms and Their Impact on Cognition, Behavior, and Function

As we delve deeper into the intricate tapestry of dementia, it's vital to understand the common symptoms and how they can drastically alter cognition, behavior, and overall function. This understanding not only aids in enhancing our approach towards care but also emboldens us with patience and empathy, which are indispensable in this journey.

Memory loss, perhaps the most recognized symptom, extends beyond mere forgetfulness. It's a deterioration that affects short-term memory initially, making it challenging for individuals to retain new information, which invariably disrupts daily activities. This can manifest in repetitive questions, misplaced belongings, or forgotten appointments, weaving a pattern of confusion and frustration not just for the person affected but also for those around them.

On the spectrum of cognitive impact, we also encounter difficulties with problem-solving and complex tasks. This could mean a once simple task like managing finances becomes a labyrinth of confusion. As decision-making skills wane, the autonomy of the individual is compromised, nudging them toward dependence on caregivers for tasks they once navigated with ease.

Language and communication bear their share of the burden too. Finding the right words becomes a Herculean task, and following conversations turns into a maze of misunderstandings. This erosion of language skills can lead to withdrawal, as the challenge of expressing thoughts becomes increasingly daunting.

Moreover, the alterations in behavior are both profound and perplexing. Mood swings, agitation, and even aggression could surface, painting a stark contrast to the individual's pre-dementia personality. These behavioral changes are not only stressful for the caregiver but also deeply distressing for the person with dementia, who may feel lost within their own emotional upheavals.

As the disease progresses, the realm of physical function does not remain untouched. Simple tasks such as dressing, bathing, and eventually eating can become insurmountable hurdles. This decline in physical capabilities necessitates a comprehensive approach to daily care, requiring patience and innovative strategies to maintain a semblance of independence.

The symptom of disorientation, both in time and space, adds another layer of complexity. Familiar surroundings turn into uncharted territories, and the concept of time becomes a puzzle, contributing to anxiety and a heightened risk of wandering.

Wandering, in itself, stands as a testament to the profound disorientation and restlessness that individuals with dementia may experience. This symptom not only poses a significant safety risk but also symbolizes the deep sense of displacement felt by those traversing the landscapes of dementia.

Moreover, sleep disturbances commonly accompany dementia, disrupting the natural rhythm of night and day. This not only affects the well-being of the person with dementia but also adds to the caregiver's load, as they navigate the nocturnal unrest and its repercussions on daytime behaviors.

The interplay between cognition, behavior, and functional abilities in dementia is complex, with each symptom intricately affecting the others. This intricate web of symptoms demands a versatile and adaptive approach to caregiving, one that evolves alongside the progression of the disease.

In managing these symptoms, creative strategies, boundless compassion, and a deep understanding of the individual's past and preferences become our most valuable tools. Adapting the living environment, establishing routines, and employing non-verbal communication can alleviate some of the challenges, allowing moments of connection and clarity to pierce through the fog of confusion.

Furthermore, it's crucial for caregivers to seek support, both for practical strategies and emotional solace. The journey of dementia, marked by its fluctuating symptoms and unpredictable progression, can be isolating. Yet, within the shared experiences of caregivers and professional guidance, lies a reservoir of strength.

Understanding the symptomatic landscape of dementia does more than just prepare us for the challenges. It opens our hearts to the nuances of the condition, fostering a caregiving approach that is both informed and empathetic. It encourages us to see beyond the symptoms, recognizing the individual still vibrant beneath the veil of dementia.

As we navigate this complex terrain, let us remember that amidst the loss, there are moments of profound connection, beauty, and understanding to be found. It's in these moments that the essence of caregiving shines through, not just as a duty, but as a deeply human act of love and devotion.

In conclusion, the symptoms of dementia and their impact on cognition, behavior, and function reshape the landscape of caregiving. Yet, through understanding, adaptability, and compassion, we can navigate this journey with grace, fostering moments of joy and connection that illuminate the path ahead.

The Emotional Impact of Witnessing Cognitive Decline

The journey of caring for a loved one with dementia is punctuated by moments of profound sadness and heartache, particularly as one witnesses the gradual erosion of the person they once knew. Seeing someone's cognitive faculties diminish – their memories fading, their grasp on language loosening, and their understanding of the world around them becoming ever more confused – is a deeply emotional experience. For caregivers, the sorrow is often twofold: grieving for the loss of the person they knew while simultaneously adjusting to the evolving needs and behaviors of the care recipient. This stage of dementia care challenges one's emotional resilience, demanding a delicate balance between acknowledging the grief and finding ways to connect and communicate within the new dynamics of the relationship. It is a test of one's ability to adapt, to find strength in vulnerability, and to seek out those fleeting moments of joy and connection amidst the sorrow. The emotional toll of witnessing cognitive decline cannot be understated, yet within this complex landscape of loss, there exists the potential for profound growth and deeper emotional connections.

Navigating Gradual Loss of Independence

As the journey into the heart of dementia continues, caregivers find themselves standing on the precipice of one of the most challenging aspects of the condition: the gradual loss of independence experienced by their loved ones. It's an inevitable part of the progression, yet knowing this does little to ease the sorrow that accompanies the observation of this decline.

Initially, the signs may be subtle – a forgotten appointment or misplaced keys. However, as time marches on, the capabilities that once defined the person you knew seem to slip away bit by bit. Activities that were undertaken with ease, now require assistance or supervision, marking a significant shift in the dynamic between caregiver and care recipient.

It's essential, in these moments, to foster an environment of patience and understanding. Resisting the inclination to complete tasks out of convenience or frustration is crucial, as it allows your loved one the dignity of endeavoring to maintain their abilities for as long as possible. This gentle balance of support and independence is not easily struck but is instrumental in navigating the psychological impact of dementia.

Adapting your communication style can significantly ease this transition. Simple, clear instructions and questions not only respect the cognitive changes occurring but also promote a sense of agency in your loved one. This adaptation in interaction lays the groundwork for a supportive atmosphere, wherein your loved one feels both valued and understood.

As tasks become more challenging, consider introducing adaptive tools that can extend independence. From specially designed kitchenware to simplify meal preparation to safety modifications in the bathroom, these adjustments can be empowering. They also serve as a subtle acknowledgment of change that respects the individual's need for autonomy.

Watching someone you care for experience this decline can be emotionally taxing. It is a period marked by grief for both the caregiver and the care recipient. Acknowledging this grief is vital, as it validates the sense of loss you are both experiencing. Engaging in open conversations about these changes, when possible, can provide a shared space for expressing feelings and fears.

During this phase, the role of the caregiver inevitably expands. Tasks previously managed by your loved one gradually fall to you, increasing both your workload and emotional burden. It's important to recognize the weight of these responsibilities and seek support when necessary. Reaching out to dementia support groups or professionals can provide not only practical advice but also a sense of community.

It is also a time to revisit care plans regularly. As independence wanes, needs evolve, demanding adjustments to daily routines and care strategies. Involving your loved one in these discussions to the extent they're able can help them retain a sense of control over their life and care.

This evolution in care needs often necessitates exploring professional help or care options. Whether it's in-home care assistance or the transition to a care facility, these decisions are incredibly difficult and fraught with emotion. Yet, they are made with your loved one's best interest at heart, aiming to provide them with the highest quality of life possible.

Maintaining your loved one's social connections is another area that requires thoughtful navigation. Encouraging visits from friends and family, when feasible, can uplift spirits and reinforce the individual's sense of self. These encounters, however, should be managed according to your loved one's comfort and capability, ensuring they remain positive experiences.

Lastly, it's crucial for caregivers to monitor their well-being during this challenging time. The demands of caregiving can be overwhelming, leading to burnout if one's health and emotional needs are neglected. Prioritizing self-care, seeking respite when needed, and embracing the support of others are key practices that sustain your ability to care for your loved one effectively.

In dealing with the gradual loss of independence, one finds themselves riding a wave of conflicting emotions - from sadness and frustration to love and determination. It requires a depth of patience, compassion, and resilience. Yet, amidst these trials, moments of profound connection and understanding can emerge, serving as poignant reminders of the enduring strength of the human spirit.

Thus, as we chart this course, it becomes clear that navigating the loss of independence is not merely about managing the decline but about embracing the journey. It's about celebrating the moments of clarity, cherishing the times of laughter, and forging a path forward that honors the dignity and worth of our loved ones as they voyage through the twilight of their independence.

In conclusion, facing the gradual loss of independence with grace necessitates a blend of practicality, compassion, and unwavering support. It asks of us to reframe our understanding of independence, recognizing that even in its loss, there are opportunities for growth, connection, and profound love. As we walk this path with our loved ones, we learn not only about the strength of the human spirit but also about the depths of our resilience and the boundless capacity of the human heart to adapt and embrace change.

The Changing Dynamics of Caregiver and Care Recipient

As we delve into the multifaceted world of dementia care, it becomes crucial to acknowledge an often subtle yet profound transition: the shifting dynamics between the caregiver and the care recipient. This dimension of care, fraught with emotional complexity and practical challenges, envelops our hearts and minds as we navigate through the journey of dementia together.

Initially, the caregiver may perceive their role as one of assistance, a helping hand in the daily tasks that become mountains for our loved ones to climb. However, as time unfurls its relentless march, the responsibilities and emotional weight burgeon, morphing from assistance to comprehensive care. This evolution, though gradual, marks a distinctive shift in the landscape of our relationship with the care recipient.

The transformation often commences with noticing the small things; perhaps it's the forgetting of names, the misplacement of keys, or the difficulty in performing routine tasks. There's an instinctive gesture to step in, to bridge the gaps that memory lapses leave behind. Yet, these instances accumulate, drawing us deeper into the role of a caregiver, a role that brings with it a gamut of emotions and decisions.

Dignity remains a cornerstone of this changing dynamic. As the ability of our loved ones to self-care diminishes, the challenge to preserve their dignity amplifies. It's a delicate dance of enabling without undermining, of offering support without usurping autonomy. This is a principle that guides us, even as we adapt to the increasing needs for assistance in dressing, eating, and personal care.

With the progression of dementia, communication transforms. The exchange of thoughts and feelings, once fluid and vibrant, becomes a landscape altered by the disease. As caregivers, our approach to communication must then shift, embracing patience and seeking understanding in new ways. This could mean learning to read non-verbal cues or finding joy and connection in shared activities when words fail us.

Amidst these changes, the role of caregiver becomes a central identity, sometimes overshadowing other aspects of our lives. This can lead to a form of grief, mourning the relationship that was, even as we adjust to the relationship that is now. It's a silent grief, perhaps, but one that earmarks this journey with profound poignancy.

Furthermore, this evolving dynamic necessitates a redefinition of independence for both the caregiver and the care recipient. For the care recipient, it's finding value and self-worth in the abilities that remain, and for the caregiver, it's the delicate balance between providing care and fostering independence, a balance that can feel like walking a tightrope.

One of the most significant aspects we face is the role reversal that often occurs. Children find themselves in the position of caring for parents, guiding them with tender authority through the days. This reversal can stir complex emotions, from resentment and guilt to an overwhelming sense of responsibility.

As we adjust to our expanding roles, it's imperative to seek support, whether through professional services, support groups, or respite care. Acknowledging that we cannot walk this path alone is not a sign of failure but of strength and wisdom. Reaching out for help allows us to sustain our own well-being, enabling us to be more present and effective caregivers.

The journey also presents moments of profound connection and unexpected joy. As the conventional forms of interaction shift, we might find new ways to connect, be it through music, art, or the simple act of sitting quietly together. These moments, fleeting yet beautiful, become treasures in the heart of changing dynamics.

It's also essential to navigate the practicalities of this dynamic with foresight and preparation. Legal and financial planning become critical, ensuring the care recipient's wishes are honored and that caregivers are empowered to make decisions. This planning, often difficult, is a necessary part of contending with the realities of dementia care.

The emotional toll on caregivers as they witness the decline of their loved ones cannot be understated. It's a path laden with challenges, requiring an inner reservoir of strength, compassion, and resilience. Self-care becomes not just advisable but essential, a lifeline amidst the tempest of caregiving.

In conclusion, the evolving dynamic between caregiver and care recipient is a testament to the complexity of human relationships, altered yet enduring in the face of dementia. It's a journey of constant adjustment, learning, and most importantly, of love. Despite the trials, it's this love that guides us, a beacon in the fog, reminding us of the deep, unbreakable bond that persists through every change and challenge.

Embracing this dynamic, understanding its nuances, and preparing for its challenges is key to navigating the path of dementia care with grace. It calls for compassion, patience, and a deep, unwavering commitment to our loved ones and to ourselves. As caregivers, it's a role we step into with trepidation, but also with hope, knowing that within the changing tides, there is the possibility of finding new depth and meaning in the relationships that define our lives.

As we turn the page, let us carry forward the lessons and insights that come from understanding and adjusting to the changing dynamics of caregiver and care recipient. It's a journey we walk together, step by step, with love as our compass and resilience as our guide.

Chapter 2:
Dementia's Ripple Effect on
Family and Relationships

The diagnosis of dementia in a family member unfolds a chapter in life filled with deep emotional complexities and stark realities. It's not just the person diagnosed who faces a litany of challenges; the entire family navigates through a turbulent sea of change. This journey, marked by its highs and lows, profoundly affects family dynamics, relationships, and roles within the household.

Witnessing a loved one's physical decline due to dementia is heart-wrenching. It's a visible reminder of the relentless nature of this condition, where each day can bring new losses. The transformation is not solely physical; cognitive changes etch deep scars in the fabric of familial connections, stirring a mix of grief, frustration, and, at times, resignation among family members.

The painful experience of role reversal is a significant aspect of dementia's impact on family relationships. Parents who were once the caregivers for their children may now find themselves dependent on those very children for daily care. This shift can stir a range of emotions, from guilt and embarrassment on the part of the parent to a sense of burden and loss on the side of the child, now caregiver.

As dementia alters family interactions, maintaining connections becomes a challenge. Behavioral changes, such as aggression or apathy, can make it difficult for family members to relate to their loved one as they once did. This transformation might leave family members grappling with feelings of loss—mourning the person they once knew, even as they stand beside them.

Coping with these behavioral changes requires patience, understanding, and a fair amount of creativity. Strategies that help maintain connections might include tapping into long-held interests or hobbies of the loved one with dementia, finding new ways to communicate, or simply being there with them, offering a comforting presence in a world that increasingly makes less sense to them.

It's crucial for families to remember they're not alone in this journey. The ripple effects of dementia touch many, and there's strength in shared experiences. Support groups, both in person and online, offer an outlet to share feelings, strategies, and support amongst those who truly understand.

Furthermore, professional help can provide a lifeline. Therapists, counselors, and dementia care specialists offer guidance and coping strategies tailored to each unique family situation, helping to navigate the rocky shores of dementia's impact on emotional and interpersonal dynamics.

Amidst these trials, there are moments of unexpected joy and profound connection. It's essential to celebrate these moments, to recognize and savor the times when the fog of dementia lifts, even if just for a moment, to reveal the loved one you remember.

Throughout this journey, families often discover an inner resilience and capacity for love that they might not have known existed. The process of caring for a loved one with dementia, while fraught with challenges, can also bring families closer, forging bonds strengthened by shared adversity.

Open communication within the family can serve as a buoy, keeping relationships afloat amid the storm. Discussing feelings openly, without judgment or blame, can help each family member process their emotions and support each other.

Adapting to new roles and responsibilities within the family is a gradual process. Flexibility, forgiveness, and understanding are key as each member finds their footing. This journey can redefine familial roles in ways that are both challenging and enriching.

It's also important to recognize when it's time to seek external help. As dementia progresses, the physical and emotional demands of caregiving can become overwhelming. Exploring options for professional care can help alleviate some of these burdens and preserve the quality of the relationship between the caregiver and the loved one.

Lastly, amidst the challenges, small victories and moments of clarity can shine brightly. Celebrating these moments, acknowledging progress and effort, can bolster the spirits of both the caregiver and the loved one with dementia.

As families traverse this complex landscape colored by dementia, the journey is undeniably hard. Yet, it is also interspersed with moments of profound beauty, deepened relationships, and the discovery of a collective strength that can weather the storm together.

In closing, the ripple effects of dementia on family and relationships are far-reaching and multifaceted. But within this journey of care, there's an opportunity for growth, for finding new depths of compassion, and for forging unbreakable bonds that endure the tempest of dementia.

Witnessing a Loved One's Physical Decline

As the shadows of dementia lengthen, witnessing a loved one's physical decline becomes an aspect of caregiving enveloped in profound sorrow and helplessness. The progression from subtle forgetfulness to significant functional losses marks a tumultuous journey, where each downturn in physical capabilities serves as a stark reminder of the relentless nature of this ailitude. Caregivers must navigate the delicate balance between fostering independence and recognizing when to step in and assist, a task that can be as heartbreaking as it is necessary. Amidst the physical transformations, the essence of the person once known seems to flicker and waver, yet it is crucial to remember that the warmth of their spirit, though obscured, is never truly extinguished. In this chapter, caregivers will find strategies to cope with their emotions and practical advice on how to adapt to their loved one's evolving needs without losing sight of the person they have always been.

The Painful Experience of Role Reversal

In the chronicles of caregiving for a loved one with dementia, the transition into the realm of role reversal presents an intricate and heartrending episode. This phase marks a seismic shift in familial roles, often feeling like the ground beneath one's feet has transformed, unsettling the known and familiar.

The world of caring for someone with dementia is fraught with challenges, not least of which is the poignant transformation in the caregiver-care recipient dynamic. As the disease progresses, the tasks and roles that once defined the individual with dementia become segments of a life they gradually leave behind. For the caregiver, particularly when they are a child of the person affected, this role reversal is not just a matter of taking on additional responsibilities—it's a profound shift in identity.

Imagine, for a moment, a daughter who once sought guidance and support from her father. Now, she finds herself managing his daily affairs, from ensuring medication compliance to handling financial matters. This reversal is not a mere change in duties; it's a profound renegotiation of their relationship. The emotional burden can be immense, for it contradicts the natural order they've both known their entire lives.

It's not just the practicalities that weigh heavily on the caregiver's shoulders; it's the emotional turmoil that accompanies watching a strong, independent parent become dependent and vulnerable. Feelings of grief and loss manifest, often long before the loved one passes, because, in many ways, the person they knew and loved is gradually fading before their eyes.

Moreover, this role reversal can trigger feelings of guilt and frustration. Guilt, because there's often an internal, nagging question of whether one is doing enough or doing it 'right.' Frustration, because despite best efforts, the progression of the disease remains relentless and unforgiving. These emotions are further compounded by the societal expectations placed on caregivers, alongside their own desires to provide care that upholds the dignity and legacy of their loved one.

In navigating this role reversal, communication becomes a double-edged sword. On one hand, it's essential for managing the practical aspects of care. On the other, it can be a source of heartache as verbal communication dwindles and caregivers strive to find new ways to connect with their loved one. These moments can bring unexpected joy in successful connection, yet also deep sorrow in the palpable sense of loss when communication fails.

Besides the emotional landscape, there's the financial and legal quagmire that often accompanies taking over a parent's affairs. It's a daunting task, replete with paperwork and decisions that carry significant consequences. This shift can feel like a loss of autonomy, not just for the person with dementia, but for the caregiver who also loses a part of their life to the ever-increasing demands of caregiving.

This role reversal often leads to a strange form of loneliness. Surrounded by people – medical professionals, fellow caregivers, perhaps even other family members – the caregiver can still feel isolated in their experience. Their world has narrowed significantly, their experiences now so profoundly different from those of their peers.

Yet, it's crucial for caregivers to seek solace in community and support groups. Sharing experiences with those who understand can alleviate the burden of loneliness. It is in these spaces that caregivers can find practical advice and emotional support, forging connections that sustain them through the tumultuous journey of caregiving.

Acceptance plays a pivotal role in managing this role reversal. Acknowledging the situation does not mean giving up hope but rather facing the reality of the condition and its implications. It is through acceptance that caregivers can find the strength to adapt, to find moments of joy amidst the sorrow, and to continue providing care with love and patience.

Patience, both with oneself and with the care recipient, becomes a cornerstone of navigating life post-role reversal. This patience is not just about enduring the challenges of the moment but about fostering an environment where the person with dementia can feel loved, supported, and valued, despite the changes in their abilities and understanding.

Within this complex emotional landscape, it's vital for caregivers to remember to care for themselves. Self-care is not selfish; it's necessary for maintaining the caregiver's well-being. This self-care might look like setting boundaries, seeking respite care, or simply allowing oneself the grace to feel and express the myriad emotions that accompany their role.

At its core, the role reversal experienced in dementia caregiving is a profound expression of love. It's a testament to the strength of the human spirit and the depths of family bonds. While fraught with challenges and sorrows, this journey is also replete with moments of unparalleled connection and profound learning.

In embracing this role reversal, caregivers embark on a tender, often heart-wrenching journey. But it's a journey that, despite its hardships, offers opportunities for growth, understanding, and deeper connection. By navigating this path with compassion, resilience, and support, caregivers can provide their loved ones with a sense of continuity, dignity, and love that endures amidst the challenges of dementia.

In conclusion, the experience of role reversal in dementia care is a multifaceted challenge. It reshapes relationships, identities, and daily life in profound ways. Yet, within this ordeal lies the possibility for profound personal and relational growth. For those walking this path, know that you are not alone, and the journey, though arduous, is paved with moments of incredible beauty and love.

How Dementia Alters Family Interactions

The emergence of dementia within the family nucleus brings about a profound transformation in its interactions, reshaping the relational terrain on which familial bonds have thrived. As cognitive faculties dim, the essence of conversation and mutual understanding undergoes a subtle, and sometimes stark, metamorphosis. Family members, in their attempts to bridge the growing chasm of communication, often find themselves oscillating between roles of caregivers and confidantes, navigating a landscape where frustration and compassion intricately intertwine. This alteration is not merely confined to the loss of shared memories but extends to the fundamental ways in which family members engage with one another. The equilibrium of giving and receiving support is disrupted, ushering in a phase where emotional resilience is both tested and fortified. Emotionally laden gestures and simplified dialogues become invaluable currencies in maintaining connections, illustrating the shift towards more elemental, yet profoundly meaningful, forms of interaction. Through this arduous journey, families are inadvertently offered a lens into the elemental facets of human connection, unearthing new depths of empathy and understanding amidst the trials posed by dementia.

Coping with Behavioral Changes and Maintaining Connections

In the realm of caring for a person with dementia, caregivers often find themselves navigating the turbulent waters of behavioral changes. This can range from mood swings and aggression to confusion and withdrawal, posing distinct challenges in maintaining emotional connections. Yet, amidst these difficulties, it's crucial to remember that heart-to-heart connections endure beyond cognitive abilities. The journey forward involves embracing patience, empathy, and innovative strategies to ensure these vital connections are not only maintained but nurtured.

Understanding the root cause of behavioral changes in dementia is a fundamental step. These alterations often result from confusion, fear, or frustration as individuals struggle to make sense of their changing world. Patience becomes an indispensable tool in these moments. Approaching your loved one with a calm demeanor and offering reassurance can make a significant difference. It's about stepping into their shoes and perceiving the world from their vantage point, which requires a deep well of empathy.

Communication plays a pivotal role in this journey. As dementia progresses, traditional forms of communication may become challenging. It's essential to adapt and find new ways to connect. This might mean relying more on non-verbal cues, such as touch, facial expressions, or body language. The power of a gentle hug or a warm smile can convey support and love in ways words cannot, establishing a profound form of connection that transcends verbal limitations.

Creating a serene environment can also help mitigate behavioral changes. This encompasses both the physical and emotional atmosphere. Ensuring the living space is clutter-free and safe can reduce incidents of confusion and agitation. Similarly, maintaining a positive emotional environment—filled with understanding, laughter, and warmth—encourages a sense of security and belonging.

Engaging in activities together that resonate with the individual's past interests offers another avenue to maintain connections. This could be as simple as listening to their favorite music, gardening together, or flipping through old photo albums. These activities can spark moments of joy and recognition, providing a bridge back to cherished memories and reinforcing the bond between caregiver and care recipient.

Adapting to the evolving needs of someone with dementia means also recognizing when to seek support. Joining a support group can provide valuable insights and strategies from those who have walked a similar path. Sharing experiences with others can also lighten the emotional load, reminding caregivers that they are not alone in their journey.

Flexibility is key. What works today might not work tomorrow, and it's okay to feel frustrated or overwhelmed at times. The important thing is to keep trying, to adapt, and to approach each day as a new opportunity for connection. Celebrating small successes, cherishing moments of clarity, and embracing periods of calm can all contribute to a sense of achievement and fulfillment for both the caregiver and the person with dementia.

Nourishing the caregiver's own well-being is equally important. Caregivers must care for themselves physically and emotionally to maintain the strength needed to support their loved ones effectively. Prioritizing self-care, finding time for personal interests, and leaning on friends, family, or professional support can help sustain the caregiver's health and enrich the quality of care provided.

Remember, the journey with dementia is unique for everyone. It's a path marked by challenges but also by moments of incredible tenderness and profound connection. Keeping a diary can be therapeutic, offering a space to express feelings, celebrate progress, and reflect on the experiences shared with the person with dementia. This not only serves to process emotions but also acts as a keepsake of the love and resilience that define the caregiving journey.

Technology can serve as an ally in maintaining connections. From simple video calls that allow visual interaction to interactive apps designed to stimulate cognitive function and memory, technology offers innovative ways to engage and connect. Even in the landscape of dementia, where cognitive abilities may wane, the desire for connection and the capacity to feel love remain intact.

At times, professional help may be necessary to address specific behavioral challenges. Consulting with healthcare professionals can provide access to strategies and medications that help manage symptoms, making it easier for caregivers to maintain a loving connection with the person with dementia.

Building a network of support is crucial. This includes friends, family, and community resources that can provide both practical and emotional support. Sharing the responsibility of care doesn't diminish the quality of the connection between the caregiver and the person with dementia. Instead, it enriches it by ensuring the caregiver's well-being and the capacity to offer consistent, loving care.

Finally, it's important to stay informed. As research into dementia progresses, new techniques and understanding continue to emerge. Staying up-to-date with the latest information can empower caregivers with new tools and perspectives to navigate the complex landscape of dementia care.

In conclusion, coping with behavioral changes and maintaining connections in the context of dementia caregiving is a multifaceted challenge. It demands patience, adaptability, and a deep reservoir of love. By focusing on understanding, communication, and the creation of a supportive environment, caregivers can find ways to connect with their loved ones in meaningful ways, ensuring that the journey, despite its difficulties, is marked by moments of joy and profound connection.

Chapter 3:
Providing Daily Care for Quality of Life

Ensuring a high quality of life for a loved one with dementia requires patience, understanding, and a little creativity. The importance of daily care cannot be overstated, as it significantly impacts the well-being of both the caregiver and the person with dementia. A cornerstone of effective care is the establishment of a consistent daily routine.

Creating a routine that is both familiar and comfortable for a person with dementia can help reduce confusion and agitation. Establishing schedules and creating step-by-step tasks for daily activities encourages a sense of independence and accomplishment. For example, a morning routine might include getting dressed, brushing teeth, and having breakfast, each broken down into manageable steps.

Visual aids prove invaluable in supporting these routines. They can range from simple pictorial day planners to notes around the home reminding your loved one of where things are kept or what tasks are to be done next. These visual cues work to gently guide and support, fostering an environment where the person can maintain as much independence as safely possible.

Meeting basic needs with compassion is another pivotal aspect of providing daily care. This includes ensuring nutritional meals, adequate hydration, and maintaining personal hygiene with dignity. Adapting to the changing needs of someone with dementia in these areas can be challenging, but there are strategies and resources available to help.

It's crucial to adapt care strategies as dementia progresses. This might mean making meals more nutritious yet easier to eat or ensuring that clothes are comfortable and simple to put on. Every person is unique, and so too will be their needs and preferences.

Consulting with healthcare professionals can provide practical support and advice for adapting care strategies. They can offer insights into nutritional needs, suggest adaptive tools for personal care, and provide guidance on maintaining physical health.

In achieving all this, caregivers are often required to become finely attuned to the evolving needs of their loved ones. This might involve regular assessments to adapt routines and care strategies as necessary. Keeping a journal can be a helpful way to track changes over time and communicate effectively with healthcare professionals.

While providing for physical needs is critical, so too is nurturing emotional wellness. Daily care is more than just attending to the physical; it's about providing comfort, ensuring safety, fostering joy, and maintaining dignity. It's the gentle touch, the patient listening, and the shared laughs that can illuminate even the cloudiest days.

Laughter, indeed, becomes a precious currency in the economy of caregiving. Finding joy in the little things, celebrating small victories, and embracing moments of connection and clarity can fortify the spirits of both caregiver and care recipient. Activities such as listening to music, looking through photo albums, or taking a leisurely walk can be simple yet effective ways to bring joy into daily routines.

Adaptability is key in providing quality daily care. What works one day may not work the next, and both caregivers and those they care for must navigate these changes together. This journey is fraught with challenges, but also filled with moments of profound beauty and deep connection.

It is also important to remember that providing quality care is not a journey one must undertake alone. Engaging family members, friends, and professional services can provide the caregiver with much-needed support and respite. It's essential to lean on available resources and recognize when to ask for help.

Part of providing quality care also involves creating opportunities for your loved one to express themselves and engage in meaningful activities. This not only enhances their quality of life but also preserves their sense of self and autonomy. Tailoring activities to match their interests and abilities can be a source of both comfort and joy.

Caring for someone with dementia is indeed a profound commitment but understanding how to provide daily care effectively can make a significant difference in the quality of life for both the caregiver and the person with dementia. Through dedication, love, and creativity, caregivers can navigate the complex realities of dementia, ensuring that their loved ones are cared for with dignity and compassion.

Finally, it's vital to step back occasionally and acknowledge the strength it takes to provide such care. Caregivers often put their own needs and well-being aside, but it's crucial to remember that taking care of oneself is also a paramount duty. Only by ensuring their own health and happiness can caregivers continue to provide the best possible care for their loved ones.

In conclusion, providing daily care with mindfulness and heart enriches the quality of life for those living with dementia. It's a journey marked by challenges, but also by the irreplaceable reward of making a meaningful difference in someone's life. Every day offers a new opportunity to provide comfort, share joy, and celebrate the genuine connection that endures despite the trials of dementia.

Creating a Consistent Daily Routine

As we journey further into the heart of providing care, one cannot overemphasize the importance of establishing a consistent daily routine for those living with dementia. Crafting a daily schedule that's both familiar and predictable can work wonders in enhancing the quality of life for your loved one. It's about weaving a tapestry of care that combines structure with flexibility, ensuring they feel secure within a framework that respects their evolving needs. From the moment the day breaks until the night's quiet settles in, each activity, meal, and rest period should serve as a gentle guide through the day, reducing confusion and anxiety. Implementing step-by-step tasks and visual aids will be discussed in subsequent sections, but it's the rhythm of routine that lays the foundation, offering an anchor in a sea of forgetfulness. Just like a lighthouse guides ships safely to shore, a well-planned routine can navigate your loved one through the day with grace and dignity, fostering a sense of accomplishment and joy in life's simple pleasures.

Establishing Schedules and Step-by-Step Tasks

In the intricate fabric of daily care for a loved one with dementia, the introduction of schedules and meticulously planned tasks serves not merely as a structure but as a beacon of normalcy in a progressively unpredictable world. Navigating this landscape requires a gentle balance between flexibility and consistency, a paradox that caregivers must embody.

Firstly, constructing a daily schedule provides a familiar framework for both caregivers and individuals with dementia. It's akin to drawing a map in a language they can understand, depicting when meals, activities, and rest periods occur. Such regularity can significantly alleviate anxiety and confusion often experienced by those with cognitive challenges.

However, the essence of effective scheduling lies in its detail. Breaking down tasks into smaller, manageable steps is crucial. For instance, instead of listing 'bathing' as a single activity, delineating it into turning on taps, adjusting the water temperature, undressing, and so on, can help in significantly reducing the overwhelm felt by your loved one.

The incorporation of visual aids alongside these tasks cannot be overstated. Simple, clear images or icons representing each step can guide an individual through their day with greater independence, fostering a sense of achievement and dignity.

Yet, while the skeleton of the schedule provides structure, its flesh and blood must be flexibility. The variable nature of dementia means that what works one day may not the next. Thus, readiness to adapt the schedule, to let go of tasks uncompleted without frustration, is a virtue that caregivers must cultivate.

In constructing this daily rhythm, caregivers are advised to prioritize the time of day when their loved one is most alert and receptive. Morning routines often work best for more complex tasks, while afternoons can be reserved for leisure and relaxation.

Eating meals at consistent times plays a significant role in this orchestration. Food not only nourishes the body but also provides social interaction and a marker of time within the day. Similarly, regular sleep schedules are paramount, as they influence mood and cognitive function.

Physical activity, woven into the day's tapestry, is essential. Be it a short walk in the garden or simple stretching exercises, movement fosters physical health and offers a change in scenery, vital for mental well-being.

Cultivating engagement through scheduled activities such as listening to music, art, or gardening can spark joy and meaningful interaction. These moments of connection, however brief, enrich the lives of everyone involved.

Moreover, integrating moments of rest and solitude is equally imperative. Caregivers must recognize the fine line between engagement and overstimulation, providing opportunities for their loved one to retreat and recharge in peace.

The inclusion of personal care tasks, approached with patience and understanding, must emphasize dignity and autonomy. Simple choices, like what to wear, can empower an individual, making these tasks less daunting.

Throughout this process, it's vital to document what works and what doesn't. Keeping a journal or log of daily activities, their successes, and challenges, can be an invaluable tool for refining the schedule and tailoring it to the evolving needs of your loved one.

Engaging other family members in this journey, sharing the responsibilities, and providing them with the schedule can foster a unified approach to care. This collective involvement not only eases the load on the primary caregiver but also enriches the support network surrounding the person with dementia.

Ultimately, the aim of establishing schedules and step-by-step tasks transcends mere organization. It's about creating a nurturing environment where moments of clarity, joy, and connection can flourish amid the fog of dementia. A testament to the enduring spirit of care, patience, and love that defines the journey of caregiving.

In closing, the dance of caregiving, with its rhythm of schedules and its melody of tasks, requires both the lead and the willingness to follow. Embracing this dance, with all its twirls and steps, can transform the caregiving experience from a burdensome chore into an expression of love, a shared journey filled with moments of unexpected beauty and grace.

Utilizing Visual Aids for Independence

In the realm of dementia care, fostering an environment where the individual can maintain as much independence as possible is paramount. It not only contributes to their sense of self but also alleviates the workload on caregivers. Among the many strategies at our disposal, visual aids stand out as a beacon of support, guiding individuals through their daily routines with an element of dignity and autonomy restored.

Much like the way a lighthouse provides direction to sailors in the murky depths, visual aids serve to navigate those living with dementia through the often confusing landscape of their daily lives. These aids come in various forms, from simple labels and color-coded systems to more elaborate pictorial guides and custom signage. Each one designed not only with the purpose of guiding but also with the intent of empowering.

Starting with something as basic as labeling, we can vastly improve the living environment for someone with dementia. Imagine cabinets and drawers clearly marked with words or pictures denoting their contents: 'clothes', 'utensils', or 'books'. This simple act can significantly reduce frustration and confusion, enabling individuals to find what they need independently.

Moreover, beyond mere labeling, color-coding items and areas in the home can further assist in navigation. Assigning a particular color to specific rooms or types of items can help in creating an intuitive understanding and memory connection. For instance, blue for bathroom-related items and red for kitchen goods simplifies the process of locating objects.

Implementing visual schedules and step-by-step task charts is another facet of utilizing visual aids effectively. A daily schedule displayed prominently in a common area, detailed with icons or pictures, assists in guiding the individual through their day. Coupled with step-by-step task charts for more complex activities, these aids can significantly enhance autonomy.

Picture-based instruction cards for common tasks, such as washing hands or preparing a simple meal, can be incredibly helpful. They break down each task into manageable steps, visually guiding the individual through the process. This not only aids in task completion but also fosters a sense of accomplishment and independence.

It is also essential to recognize the emotional benefits of visual aids. The frustration stemming from the inability to perform previously simple tasks can be overwhelming. Providing tools that mitigate this can contribute greatly to emotional well-being. There's a certain sense of normalcy and comfort that can be reclaimed when an individual is able to navigate their day with less assistance.

Custom signage within the home, tailored to the specific needs of the individual, can be a game-changer. Large, clear signs that direct to the bathroom, bedroom, or living room can ease the stress of orientation. For someone struggling with memory issues, these signs are a helping hand in a world that increasingly feels unfamiliar.

Additionally, integrating technology as a visual aid, through apps or digital devices designed for dementia care, can introduce another layer of assistance. These digital aids can provide reminders, entertainment, and even social connection, all through user-friendly, visually-based interfaces.

When implementing visual aids, it's crucial to involve the person with dementia in the process, as much as their condition allows. This involvement ensures that the aids are truly beneficial and tailored to their unique preferences and needs. It's about enhancing their life, not just imposing solutions.

The design of visual aids should be clear, with minimal visual clutter, and use large, easy-to-read fonts. This consideration makes it easier for individuals with visual impairments or cognitive challenges to understand and use them. The goal is to make these aids as accessible and unambiguous as possible.

It's also worth noting that the effectiveness of visual aids may evolve over time. As dementia progresses, the types and complexity of aids that are helpful may change. Regularly assessing and adjusting these tools is key to maintaining their effectiveness and ensuring they continue to support independence.

In tandem with other strategies for dementia care, such as creating a consistent daily routine and adapting the living space for safety and ease of use, visual aids can significantly improve the quality of life. They offer a way to bridge the gap between the individual's capability and their environment, enabling them to engage more fully in their world.

Ultimately, the use of visual aids in dementia care is a testament to the power of seeing. In a world where words can become lost and memories fade, the visual remains a strong anchor. Through thoughtful implementation of these tools, caregivers can offer a lifeline to those they care for, anchoring them back to a sense of independence and self.

The journey of caregiving is marked by challenges, but it's also filled with opportunities to make meaningful impacts on our loved ones' lives. By utilizing visual aids for independence, we can turn daily routines into a series of small victories, each one restoring a piece of autonomy to the person in our care. It's a nuanced balance of support and empowerment, both essential ingredients in the complex recipe of dementia care.

Meeting Basic Needs with Compassion

Providing for someone with dementia means stepping into their world and understanding their needs, often without them having to articulate anything. It requires a level of empathy and patience that goes beyond the ordinary. Meeting basic needs with compassion lies at the heart of ensuring quality of life for those on this challenging journey. Nutrition, hydration, and hygiene might seem like simple components of daily care, but for individuals with dementia, these areas need special consideration and approach.

When addressing the issue of nutrition, one must remember that taste preferences and eating habits can significantly change. For some, the flavors they once loved might now seem unappealing, or they may struggle to recognize certain foods. In such cases, it's essential to remain flexible and patient, offering a variety of choices and focusing on nutrient-dense foods to ensure they receive the necessary nourishment. Incorporating their preferences, no matter how unconventional they might seem, becomes a cornerstone of compassionate care.

Similarly, ensuring adequate hydration presents its own set of challenges. Individuals with dementia may not always remember to drink water or might not feel thirst in the same way they once did. Keeping them hydrated requires regular prompts or incorporating foods with high water content into their diet. Offering a cup of water or their favorite drink, perhaps in a special cup they are fond of, can make a difference in their intake.

Hygiene is another critical aspect that requires a compassionate approach. With the progression of dementia, tasks like bathing or brushing teeth can become confusing or frightening experiences. It's crucial to establish a routine that makes these tasks as comfortable and dignified as possible. Creating a calm environment, ensuring privacy, and explaining each step in a reassuring tone can help alleviate stress and anxiety associated with personal care.

Adapting to these evolving needs doesn't just stop at the physical level. Emotional connection plays a significant role in providing care. Engaging in conversations, even if they are one-sided, and maintaining eye contact can convey a sense of security and love. It's about making them feel seen and valued, no matter where they are in their dementia journey.

Moreover, adapting the physical environment to suit these needs is paramount. Clearing pathways, ensuring easy access to snacks and drinks, and safety-proofing the bathroom can promote a sense of independence and confidence in their abilities. Sometimes, simple adjustments can lead to significant improvements in their daily living experience.

Consulting with professionals can also offer strategies and insights tailored to the individual's specific needs. Dietitians, occupational therapists, and dementia care specialists can provide valuable advice on creating a care plan that addresses nutrition, hydration, and hygiene in ways that respect the dignity and preferences of the person.

Implementing visual aids is another method to support daily care routines. Labeling cabinets with pictures of their contents or posting reminders to drink water can help those in the earlier stages of dementia maintain some level of independence. These small acts of compassion can significantly enhance their quality of life.

In moments of frustration or refusal, which are not uncommon, it's important for caregivers to remain patient and not take these reactions personally. Understanding that these responses are part of the disease can help caregivers approach such situations with empathy and find alternative ways to meet their loved one's needs.

Equally, recognizing when to step back and offer choices can empower those with dementia. Even simple decisions, such as choosing between two outfits or what to eat for breakfast, can provide a sense of control and normalcy in their lives. These moments of autonomy are precious and need to be nurtured with compassion and sensitivity.

It's also beneficial to celebrate small successes and joyful moments together. Whether it's a successful mealtime or a positive response to hygiene care, acknowledging these moments can lift the spirits of both the caregiver and the one receiving care. It serves as a reminder of the love and commitment that guides the caregiving journey.

Throughout this process, caregivers must also practice self-compassion. Recognizing the emotional toll that caregiving can take and allowing oneself grace during difficult moments is essential. Seeking support, whether through support groups or respite care, can provide the necessary rest and rejuvenation to continue offering compassionate care.

In the end, meeting basic needs with compassion is about more than just sustaining life; it's about enriching it. It's about facing each day with a heart full of kindness, a mind equipped with knowledge, and arms ready to provide comfort. This compassionate approach not only enhances the quality of life for those with dementia but also brings immeasurable rewards to the caregivers themselves.

Caregiving in the landscape of dementia is a journey of love, patience, and resilience. By meeting basic needs with compassion, caregivers can navigate this path with grace, ensuring their loved ones feel supported, understood, and cherished every step of the way.

Adapting Care for Nutrition, Hydration, and Hygiene

As we continue to navigate the intricacies of providing daily care for our loved ones with dementia, it becomes imperative to hone our focus on three fundamental aspects: nutrition, hydration, and hygiene. These elements are critical in maintaining not only the physical health but also the overall well-being of individuals living with this condition.

When it comes to nutrition, understanding and responding to the changing needs and preferences of our loved ones can be challenging. Appetites may fluctuate, and familiar foods might suddenly become unappealing or difficult to consume. It's essential, therefore, to approach mealtime with flexibility and patience. Offering smaller, more frequent meals can be an effective strategy, as can the inclusion of nutrient-dense foods that are easier to eat, such as smoothies or soups.

Hydration follows closely in importance, yet it can be easily overlooked. Dementia can impair a person's ability to recognize thirst, leading to dehydration if not carefully monitored. Keeping a variety of beverages available, and encouraging sips throughout the day, can help ensure adequate fluid intake. Sometimes, offering water in different forms, such as ice pops or gelatin, might be more appealing and can be an enjoyable way to increase hydration.

The task of maintaining personal hygiene presents its set of challenges. Cognitive impairments can make the routine of bathing, brushing teeth, and other personal care tasks confusing or frustrating. Dignity and respect are paramount in these situations. Establishing a predictable routine can reduce anxiety and make these necessary activities more comforting. It may also be helpful to use products designed for sensitive skin or specialized dental care items that simplify oral hygiene.

One cannot underestimate the importance of engaging the senses during meals and hygiene routines. Using brightly colored plates can make food more visually appealing and might stimulate appetite. Similarly, incorporating familiar scents into bathing rituals can evoke memories and make the experience more pleasant.

In dealing with feeding difficulties, especially in later stages, consider consulting a speech therapist for advice on making swallowing safer and more comfortable. They might recommend specific utensils or techniques to facilitate easier eating, thereby reducing the risk of choking or aspiration.

Constipation is an often-overlooked concern that can significantly impact comfort and health. A diet rich in fiber, alongside proper hydration, can aid in promoting regular bowel movements. Gentle, regular physical activity, as much as possible, can also support digestive health.

Clothing choices can influence a person's ability to manage personal care tasks independently. Opt for garments that are easy to put on and remove, such as those with Velcro closures or elastic waistbands. This consideration not only supports autonomy but also preserves dignity.

While it's crucial to support physical needs, we mustn't overlook the emotional and psychological impact of these intimate care tasks. Engaging in gentle conversation, using humor appropriately, and maintaining a calm and reassuring presence can all contribute to a positive experience.

For those individuals who may resist care, especially in tasks like bathing or changing clothes, it's worth considering the timing and environment. Sometimes, a different time of day or a warmer room can make all the difference in their comfort and willingness to participate.

Sleep hygiene also plays a vital role in overall health. Ensuring a comfortable, quiet sleeping environment, and a consistent bedtime routine can promote better sleep. Avoiding stimulating activities or foods and drinks late in the day can also help in this regard.

It's essential for caregivers to keep detailed records of their loved one's eating habits, fluid intake, and bowel movements. These logs can be invaluable in identifying patterns or changes that may indicate a need for medical attention or dietary adjustments.

Finally, don't hesitate to reach out for professional help when needed. Dietitians can provide personalized guidance on nutrition, while occupational therapists can offer strategies to simplify daily care tasks. Remember, you're not alone in this journey, and seeking support is a sign of strength and commitment to your loved one's well-being.

Embarking on this path requires patience, creativity, and a deep reservoir of compassion. Adaptability is key. What works today may need reevaluation tomorrow. Celebrate the small victories, and be gentle with yourself through the challenges.

In conclusion, providing care in the realms of nutrition, hydration, and hygiene is a dynamic and evolving process. By staying informed, flexible, and responsive to our loved ones' needs, we can ensure they receive the care and dignity they deserve.

Consulting Professionals for Practical Support

In navigating the demanding journey of caregiving for a loved one with dementia, it becomes crucial to seek out and consult professionals for practical support. This pursuit not only enlightens the path ahead but also alleviates the burden that often weighs heavily upon the caregiver's shoulders. It's in this vein that we explore the paramount importance of aligning oneself with experts in various fields to garner support that's both pragmatic and tailored to your unique circumstance.

First and foremost, engaging with a medical professional who specializes in geriatric care or neurology can offer significant insight into the condition itself, its trajectory, and the management of symptoms. Such expertise is indispensable, not only for the individual with dementia but also for the caregiver, equipping them with a comprehensive understanding of what to expect and how to prepare for the journey ahead.

Another critical avenue for professional support is found in the realm of occupational therapy. Occupational therapists can provide practical strategies to enable individuals with dementia to maintain as much independence as possible. From adapting the living environment to enhance safety and functionality to recommending specific activities that stimulate cognitive function and motor skills, their guidance is invaluable in fostering a sense of normalcy and autonomy for your loved one.

Similarly, consulting a nutritionist or dietician who is familiar with dementia care can be profoundly beneficial. As dietary needs shift and challenges with eating and drinking emerge, these professionals offer tailored advice to ensure that nutritional needs are met in a manner that is both appealing and manageable for someone with cognitive challenges.

Moreover, speech and language therapists can play a pivotal role, particularly as communication barriers arise. They provide tools and techniques to facilitate communication, making the process less frustrating for both the caregiver and the individual with dementia. Their interventions can also support swallowing issues, thereby preventing potential complications related to nutrition and hydration.

Physical therapists, too, are instrumental in the caregiving journey. They assist in developing exercise programs that are suited to the individual's current capabilities, with an eye toward enhancing strength, balance, and mobility. Such programs can significantly contribute to the overall well-being of your loved one, reducing the risk of falls and other physical complications.

Seeking support from legal and financial advisors knowledgeable about elder care is equally important. They can provide guidance on matters such as estate planning, advance directives, and navigating public benefits, ensuring that the caregiver is well-prepared to make informed decisions regarding the legal and financial aspects of care.

For those moments when the emotional and psychological toll becomes particularly heavy, mental health professionals, including psychologists and counselors who specialize in caregiving and dementia, can offer a much-needed respite. Through counseling and therapy, they provide strategies to manage stress, cope with grief, and maintain one's mental health.

Another vital aspect of caregiving is understanding and managing medication. Pharmacists and geriatric pharmacologists can be consulted to ensure that medications are optimized to improve symptoms while minimizing side effects, thus enhancing the quality of life for the individual with dementia.

Social workers specializing in elder care are also key allies in this journey. They can connect caregivers with community resources, support groups, and services designed to assist both the caregiver and the loved one. Their knowledge can pave the way for accessing additional support such as respite care, in-home assistance, and day programs tailored to individuals with dementia.

In certain instances, enlisting the services of professional care coordinators or case managers can prove invaluable. These professionals can oversee the comprehensive care needs of the individual, coordinating between various healthcare providers and services to ensure a seamless care experience.

Furthermore, joining forces with hospice care professionals as the disease progresses can provide both comfort and dignity to your loved one in the final stages of dementia. These experts offer palliative care, addressing physical symptoms, and providing emotional and spiritual support to the family.

In addition to these professionals, it can be beneficial to consult with experts in adaptive technologies and home modifications. These individuals can recommend products and modifications to create a safer, more accessible home environment, thereby promoting independence and preventing accidents.

Lastly, it is crucial to remember that while the journey of caregiving for a loved one with dementia is undoubtedly challenging, it does not have to be navigated alone. By consulting with a spectrum of professionals, caregivers can arm themselves with the knowledge, tools, and support necessary to provide compassionate care while also preserving their own well-being.

In sum, consulting professionals for practical support encompasses a multidisciplinary approach, embracing the medical, psychological, legal, and day-to-day practical facets of caregiving. It underscores a proactive stance, advocating for the highest possible quality of life for both the caregiver and the individual with dementia. Embracing this collaborative approach can make all the difference in traversing this complex and tender journey.

Chapter 4:
Crafting a Safe and Supportive
Home Environment

As caregivers enter the fold of adjusting their homes, it's imperative to pivot toward crafting an environment that is not only physically safe but also emotionally nurturing for individuals with dementia. The essence of crafting such a space lies in understanding the unique challenges and hazards that might not be evident at first glance. This chapter delves into the practical aspects of designing an enabling environment that fosters a sense of independence while safeguarding against potential risks.

Creating a dementia-friendly home begins with a thorough assessment of the living space. This means identifying areas that may pose risks such as slippery floors, sharp corners, or difficult-to-navigate furniture arrangements. One of the first steps is simplifying the environment to reduce confusion and anxiety. This can include removing excess clutter, ensuring adequate lighting, and labeling cabinets and rooms with clear, large text or color-coded signs to help with navigation and identification.

Another component of ensuring safety is home proofing. Similar to baby-proofing, home proofing for a person with dementia involves adding locks or alarms to doors and windows to prevent wandering, securing rugs to the floor to minimize tripping hazards, and installing grab bars in the bathroom to assist with mobility. Home proofing is a continuous process that adapts to the evolving needs of the care recipient.

The challenge of wandering, a common behavior in later stages of dementia, requires particular attention. Caregivers might consider installing door alarms or GPS tracking devices and registering their loved one with local police departments as part of a safe return program. It's not just about preventing wandering but ensuring the quick and safe return of the individual should they wander.

On the emotional front, creating a supportive home goes beyond physical modifications. It's about fostering an environment where the individual feels secure, valued, and loved. This includes incorporating familiar objects and personal items into the decor to promote a sense of belonging and continuity.

Music and pets can also play a significant role in creating a nurturing atmosphere. Studies have shown that music, particularly songs from the individual's youth, can evoke memories and promote relaxation. Similarly, the presence of a calm and friendly pet can provide companionship and comfort.

Engaging the senses is another strategy to enhance the home environment. This can involve using essential oils for calming effects, tactile objects like soft blankets or stress balls to engage the hands, and visual stimuli such as family photos displayed prominently.

Communication within this adapted space is key. Caregivers should strive for clear, positive communication, utilizing short, simple sentences and maintaining eye contact. This contributes to a supportive environment by reducing potential frustrations and misunderstandings.

The kitchen and dining area also require special attention. Since nutrition is paramount, caregivers may need to adapt the kitchen to encourage independence while ensuring safety. This could include accessible snacks that are easy to open, adaptive utensils for easier grip, and clear, simple instructions for small meals.

In the realm of technology, smart home devices can offer support and enhance safety. Automated lights can help prevent falls at night, while smart locks can control access to dangerous areas or prevent wandering. Voice-activated assistants can offer reminders for medication or appointments, acting as an aid for both the caregiver and the individual with dementia.

Beyond the structural modifications and technological aids, the emotional well-being of the person with dementia is paramount. Initiatives such as creating a 'memory box' filled with photos and mementos can help in sparking conversations and reminiscing about pleasant memories, contributing to a sense of identity and self.

Collaboration with healthcare professionals can further refine the home environment. Occupational therapists, in particular, can offer insights into specific adaptations that can promote independence for as long as possible. They can suggest modifications that might not be obvious to someone not trained in dementia care, ensuring the home is as safe and supportive as it can be.

Lastly, the concept of a supportive home is not static; it evolves. As dementia progresses, the needs of the person will change, and so must their environment. Regular reassessment of the living space and adaptability in the approach to care are key to providing the best possible support.

In crafting a safe and supportive home environment for a loved one with dementia, caregivers embark on a journey filled with challenges but also opportunities for deep connection and fulfillment. Through thoughtful modifications and a steadfast commitment to nurturing the emotional and physical well-being of the individual, caregivers can profoundly impact their loved one's quality of life.

This chapter has emphasized the importance of balancing safety with emotional support, considering not just the physical adaptations needed but also the sensory and emotional aspects that contribute to a truly supportive home. It's a testament to the fact that with the right approaches and adaptations, caregivers can create a haven that supports their loved one's journey through dementia with dignity and love.

Designing an Enabling Space

Transforming a home into an enabling space for a loved one with dementia is not only a necessity but an ongoing act of love. It's about creating an environment that supports independence, ensures safety, and nurtures well-being. The essence of a well-designed space lies in its ability to adapt to the evolving needs of someone living with dementia, fostering a sense of normalcy and security amidst the changes they experience.

Firstly, consider the overall layout of your home. It should facilitate easy navigation and minimize the risks of falls, which are common concerns. Removing clutter and ensuring clear paths in and around the house can significantly reduce these risks. It's also beneficial to assess the lighting, as adequate illumination can help in reducing confusion and enhancing visibility, particularly during the evening and night when visibility decreases.

Safety adjustments are paramount and often involve simple measures such as installing grab bars in strategic locations like bathrooms and along staircases, and ensuring that rugs are secured to prevent slips. The bedroom, often overlooked, deserves attention too, with considerations for an adjustable bed and a night light to guide the way during nocturnal awakenings.

In the kitchen, simplicity and security should dictate the arrangement. Appliances that automatically shut off and cabinets that can be locked if necessary help prevent accidents. Labels and easy-to-use gadgets can empower individuals to participate in meal preparation, fostering a sense of accomplishment and normalcy.

Bathrooms present unique challenges but also opportunities for adaptive strategies. Non-slip mats, raised toilet seats, and walk-in showers enhance safety. Color contrasts between towels, toilet seats, and the floor can help delineate different areas, aiding those with visual spatial challenges.

Creating a supportive living environment also means considering cognitive aids. Large clocks, calendars, and photo albums can be strategically placed around the house to help orient your loved one to time and place. Color-coding or labeling household items can assist in their identification, promoting independence.

Personal spaces should be tailored to reflect the person's history and preferences, incorporating familiar and cherished items. These elements can anchor them to their identity and past, providing comfort amidst confusion. A well-curated space can offer non-verbal cues about routines and help in locating personal items.

The importance of outdoor spaces should not be underestimated. A secured garden or a safely enclosed patio can offer a vital connection with nature and the outside world. Such spaces should be easy to navigate and provide restful areas with seating to enjoy the outdoors.

Technology, too, plays a critical role in designing an enabling environment. From simple devices like automatic night lights to more sophisticated systems like GPS trackers for those who wander, technology can provide solutions that reinforce safety and support autonomy.

Despite these adaptations, the home should remain a place of warmth and familiarity. The balance between safety features and a homely atmosphere is delicate but achievable. The ultimate goal is to make the home a sanctuary that supports a sense of belonging and well-being for the person with dementia.

Engaging your loved one in the redesigning process, as much as possible, can provide valuable insights into their preferences and comfort. While not all their desires may be feasible, involving them can ensure that the space not only meets their needs but also reflects their personality.

Professional advice from occupational therapists or dementia care experts can be invaluable in identifying specific adjustments and innovations that cater to the unique requirements of your loved one. Their expertise can guide you in making informed decisions that enhance functionality and safety.

Adapting your home is an evolving process that mirrors the progression of dementia. Regular reassessments of the living space are essential to meet the changing needs of your loved one. Flexibility and creativity in approach allow for adjustments that can make significant differences in their quality of life.

Lastly, remember that every change made is a step towards creating an enabling environment. It's about empowering your loved one to live as independently and safely as possible. It's a journey made together, with patience and love, as you both navigate the complexities of dementia.

In conclusion, designing an enabling space is a multifaceted endeavor that requires thoughtful consideration of physical, cognitive, and emotional needs. It's a labor of love that not only enhances safety but also promotes independence, dignity, and quality of life for individuals with dementia. By carefully crafting such an environment, caregivers can offer their loved ones a supportive and nurturing home that anticipates and accommodates the challenges posed by dementia.

Home Proofing and Simplification Strategies

In the labyrinth of dementia care, crafting a space that aligns with the evolving needs of a loved one is a gesture of profound understanding and respect. It's about transforming the home into a sanctuary of safety and simplicity, where every corner whispers reassurance, and each object serves a purpose.

Starting this journey, it's essential to view the home through the lens of someone living with dementia. What might appear benign to us can become a source of confusion or harm to them. Thus, the first step is a thorough walk-through of your living space, noting potential hazards and areas of difficulty. Look for trip hazards like loose rugs, clutter that might impede navigation, or furniture that could become an obstacle.

Lighting plays a crucial role in the comfort and safety of those with cognitive challenges. Ensure that the home is brightly lit, with natural light wherever possible. This isn't merely for aesthetic pleasure, but to help distinguish between day and night, reducing confusion and aiding in navigation. At night, consider installing motion-sensor lights to guide the way to the bathroom or kitchen without overwhelming with bright, constant lighting.

Simplification goes beyond decluttering; it involves rethinking the living environment. For instance, complex appliances can become sources of frustration or danger. Opt for simple, user-friendly devices that don't challenge but assist. A kettle with an automatic shut-off, a microwave with basic functions, or a telephone with preset numbers can foster independence while ensuring safety.

The challenge of recognition in dementia can turn even familiar settings into mazes. Use labels and signs on doors, cabinets, and drawers to remind your loved one what can be found within. Pictures can be particularly useful, serving as visual cues for those who struggle with reading or word recognition.

Adapting spaces to reduce confusion is also a key. For example, mirrors can sometimes cause distress if the individual doesn't recognize their reflection. Covering these or removing them from critical areas can prevent unnecessary anxiety. Similarly, patterns on wallpapers or upholstery that might appear to move or change can be disorienting, so opting for solid colors is favorable.

Consider safety in every aspect of home life, including the bathroom. Install grab bars near the toilet and in the shower or tub to prevent falls. Non-slip mats inside and outside the bathing area are essential. If traditional showers or tubs pose too high a risk, consider a walk-in model that reduces the need to step over a high edge.

In the kitchen, safety measures include locking cabinets that contain potentially dangerous items such as cleaning supplies or sharp tools. A stove with an automatic shut-off feature can mitigate the risk of burns or fires. Always ensure that fire extinguishers and smoke detectors are in working order and that your loved one is familiar with an evacuation plan in case of emergencies.

The aspect of wandering, a common behavior in later stages of dementia, demands preemptive planning. Secure your home by installing alarms on doors and windows that alert you when they're opened. Consider a GPS device or wearable technology that can help track your loved one's location should they wander away.

Don't underestimate the importance of creating a therapeutic environment. Incorporating elements that spark joy, memories, or a sense of calm can have a profound effect. This can mean displaying photographs of family and friends, playing favorite music, or maintaining a small garden.

Accessibility adjustments, such as levers instead of knobs for doors and faucets, can ease the physical strain and promote independence. Furniture should be sturdy and easy to navigate around, with clear paths in every room to avoid confusion and falls.

Maintaining continuity and familiarity is comforting. Keep the home layout as consistent as possible, and avoid unnecessary changes that could lead to disorientation. When alterations are necessary, introduce them gradually, and provide plenty of reassurance and guidance.

Lastly, involve your loved one in the process as much as possible. Giving them a voice in the decisions about their living environment respects their autonomy and can help them feel more at ease with the changes. This collaboration, though it may require patience, strengthens bonds and fosters trust.

In conclusion, home proofing and simplification are not just tasks; they are acts of love and empathy. They require us to step into the shoes of those we care for, to anticipate their needs, and to make their world as safe and understandable as we can. While dementia may steal many things, it cannot take away the sanctuary of a thoughtfully arranged home.

Remember, these strategies are not exhaustive, and every individual's needs will evolve. Stay observant, flexible, and compassionate. As your loved one's world changes, so too will your strategies for maintaining their comfort and safety. But in each step, know that you're creating a space not only of safety but of dignity and respect.

Navigating the Challenge of Wandering

Wandering is a common and complex behavior observed in individuals with dementia, presenting an array of challenges for caregivers tasked with ensuring their loved one's safety. This chapter will delve into tactics and strategies caregivers can employ to address the wandering behavior effectively, mitigating risks while respecting the autonomy and dignity of those in their care.

The impulse to wander can stem from various needs or desires, such as the search for something familiar, a response to basic needs such as hunger or thirst, or an attempt to satisfy a once routine habit like going to work. Understanding the root cause can be instrumental in managing this behavior, and in some cases, can guide the caregiver in preventing the occurrence of wandering.

Creating a safe and supportive home environment is the first step in addressing wandering. This encompasses a range of strategies from home proofing to simplification techniques designed to make the living space not only secure but also comforting and navigable for someone with cognitive challenges.

Technology can play a pivotal role in managing a loved one's propensity to wander. Various forms of wearable GPS devices and home monitoring systems can provide peace of mind to caregivers by ensuring that even if wandering occurs, the individual can be located and assisted promptly.

Redirecting the focus of someone with dementia can be an effective strategy when signs of restlessness or wandering behavior begin to surface. Engaging in a distraction that is both meaningful and enjoyable for the person can divert their attention away from wandering to a more secure and engaging activity.

Developing a daily routine and adhering to it can help reduce instances of wandering. A structured schedule provides a sense of stability and predictability, which can be comforting to individuals with dementia, thereby diminishing their need to seek out the familiar in unsafe ways.

Communication plays a significant role in handling wandering behavior. It's crucial for caregivers to maintain a calm demeanor and adopt a reassuring tone when interacting with their loved one. This approach not only aids in de-escalating potential wandering situations but also fosters a nurturing care environment.

In cases where wandering leads a person outside the safety of their home, having a plan in place is critical. This includes notifying neighbors and local authorities about the individual's condition, so they can better assist if they find the person disoriented or lost.

Another practical step is ensuring the individual carries identification or wears medical alert jewelry that indicates they have dementia. This simple measure can be a lifeline in situations where they might wander away from their known surroundings.

Design modifications to the home environment, such as installing locks out of the line of sight and utilizing door alarms, can deter wandering. Additionally, creating a designated safe zone within the home where the individual can move freely without risk can offer a compromise between safety and autonomy.

It's also helpful to encourage physical activity and social engagement within safe boundaries. Regular exercise and interaction can satisfy the urge for movement and exploration in a controlled manner, potentially reducing the frequency of wandering.

Professional guidance from healthcare providers who specialize in dementia care can offer insights tailored to the unique needs of the individual. Such expertise can enrich a caregiver's arsenal of strategies for managing wandering, providing both preventive and reactive solutions.

Support groups and communities of fellow caregivers are invaluable resources for sharing experiences and tips related to wandering. Learning from the collective wisdom of those who have navigated similar challenges can inspire innovative solutions and foster a sense of solidarity.

Ultimately, the objective in managing wandering is to balance safety concerns with the individual's need for independence and exploration. Recognizing wandering as a communication of an unmet need or desire enables caregivers to adopt a compassionate, informed approach to safeguarding their loved ones.

In closing, while the challenge of wandering may seem daunting, it can be navigated with patience, understanding, and the strategic application of the resources and techniques shared in this chapter. Caregivers equipped with this knowledge can create an environment that minimizes the risks associated with wandering while enhancing the quality of life for those in their care.

Chapter 5:
Caring for Yourself as a Caregiver

In the labyrinth of emotions and responsibilities that envelop the role of caregiving, it's easy to overlook the one person who is the lynchpin in this entire endeavor: the caregiver. Amidst the challenges and the relentless demands of caring for a loved one with dementia, prioritizing your own well-being is not just beneficial; it's absolutely crucial. This chapter will delve into strategies and insights on how to adequately care for yourself while you give care, ensuring sustainability and well-being in this arduous journey.

Prioritizing self-care is not a luxury—it's a necessity. Remember, you can't pour from an empty cup. To effectively look after someone else, you must first ensure that you are looked after. This means not only attending to your physical health but also nurturing your emotional and psychological well-being. It involves acknowledging the weight of your responsibilities and understanding that seeking respite and external help isn't a sign of weakness, but of wisdom.

Embracing respite care and seeking external assistance are essential strategies in self-care. Respite care provides you with the opportunity to take a break, recharge your batteries, and return to caregiving with renewed energy and perspective. This break can be anything from a few hours to several days, depending on your needs and situation. Exploring options for professional in-home care, adult day care programs, or short-term residential care facilities can offer the support you need to take this well-deserved respite.

Equally crucial is the effort to keep your personal connections alive. Maintaining friendships and nurturing relationships outside of your caregiving duties can provide you with valuable emotional support and a much-needed outlet for relaxation and rejuvenation. Let these connections be a reminder of your identity beyond your role as a caregiver—a space where you can be yourself, unburdened and unfettered.

Leaning on support networks and seeking professional help when needed can significantly mitigate the isolating experience of caregiving. Connecting with others who understand what you're going through can be incredibly validating and empowering. Whether it's through local support groups or online communities, finding a platform to share your experiences, challenges, and victories can lighten your emotional load.

Moreover, exploring counseling and support group options can provide you with strategies to cope with the stress and emotional toll of caregiving. Professional guidance can offer not just practical advice but also a safe space to process your feelings and experiences. It's a profound act of self-care to acknowledge when the burden feels too heavy and to seek professional help to carry it.

Emphasizing the importance of self-care reflects a deeper understanding of the interdependency between the caregiver and the care recipient. Caring for yourself enables you to provide the best possible care for your loved one. It's a balance that ensures both your well-being and theirs. This balance involves finding moments of joy and relaxation amid the caregiving tasks, recognizing and celebrating small victories, and permitting yourself the grace to acknowledge the challenges without being consumed by them.

Initiating a routine for your well-being that can coexist with your caregiving duties is another step towards achieving this balance. Incorporating simple practices like mindfulness, short walks, or reading can significantly contribute to your mental and emotional health. These activities don't have to be time-consuming or elaborate; they just need to be consistent and meaningful to you.

Maintaining your physical health is also critical. It's easy to neglect physical exercise and proper nutrition when you're consumed by caregiving responsibilities. Yet, ensuring that you're getting enough rest, eating well, and staying active is fundamental to your capacity to care for someone else. Consider these activities as non-negotiable appointments on your calendar, akin to any important caregiving task.

Moreover, establishing clear boundaries is essential in managing the demanding role of a caregiver. Understanding and communicating your limits, both to yourself and others, can prevent burnout. It's important to recognize that saying no or delegating tasks does not equate to failure. Rather, it's an essential skill in sustaining your health and well-being.

One of the most significant aspects of self-care is the practice of self-compassion. Being kind to yourself, forgiving yourself for perceived shortcomings, and understanding that you are doing your best in an incredibly difficult situation is crucial. Allow yourself the grace to feel overwhelmed, to grieve, and to seek joy in the midst of it all.

In every step of your caregiving journey, remember that caring for yourself is not a detour from caring for your loved one. Instead, it's an integral part of the caregiving process. It ensures that you have the strength, resilience, and health to provide the care that your loved one needs. It's a testament to the understanding that, to give care is also to receive it—to acknowledge that in the intricate dance of caregiving, the caregiver's well-being is as paramount as that of the care recipient.

Lastly, keep in mind that seeking and accepting help does not diminish the love and dedication you have for your loved one. It amplifies it. By caring for yourself, you're ensuring that you can be there for your loved one, not just in presence but in spirit, energy, and strength. This journey is undeniably tough, but through self-care, resilience, and support, it can also be incredibly rewarding.

In conclusion, caring for yourself while you care for a loved one with dementia is a complex, yet wholly necessary endeavor. It demands bravery to prioritize your well-being, wisdom to seek support, and compassion to embrace self-care as an integral part of your caregiving role. Through these practices, you not only sustain your health and happiness but also enhance your ability to provide compassionate, effective care for your loved one. Remember, to care for yourself is not just an act of self-love—it's an essential component of loving someone else.

Prioritizing Self-Care for Sustainability

In the realm of caregiving, it's easy to lose sight of one's own well-being amidst the tireless efforts to support a loved one facing dementia. Yet, it is precisely in this selfless act that the necessity for self-care becomes paramount, for the sustainability of both the caregiver and the care receiver depends upon it. Acknowledging the gravity of this role, the act of caring for oneself isn't just advisable; it becomes a critical component of the caregiving journey. Engaging in regular, meaningful self-care practices not only replenishes your physical and emotional reserves but also sharpens your abilities to provide compassionate, effective care. From setting aside time for personal hobbies and interests to ensuring proper rest and nutrition, making self-care a non-negotiable part of your routine keeps burnout at bay. Moreover, seeking respite care and embracing the support of a community can significantly lighten the load, allowing moments of pause and reflection. In nurturing oneself, you not only safeguard your health but also model the compassion and care that define your role, ensuring a more sustainable path forward in the caregiving journey.

Embracing Respite and External Help

As we navigate the winding path that is caregiving, it becomes evident that tending to a loved one with dementia is not a journey one should embark on alone. The complexities and demands of caregiving necessitate a pause, a moment of rest, and the acceptance of external support. This section delves into the essential nature of respite and the invaluable assistance external help can provide.

In the realm of caregiving, the concept of respite is not merely a luxury but a requirement. To replenish one's strength and sustain the quality of care, stepping away momentarily from the responsibilities of caregiving is crucial. Respite can take many forms, from a few hours spent in the company of books or nature to a more extended break facilitated by professional respite services.

Seeking professional help is a testament to the caregiver's strength, not a sign of weakness. Various forms of external assistance, ranging from home health aides to adult day care services, can provide not only practical support but also emotional and psychological relief. Leveraging these resources allows caregivers to maintain their well-being while ensuring that their loved ones receive the best possible care.

Finding the right type of external help requires research and assessment of the specific needs of both the caregiver and the person with dementia. Home care services, for instance, offer tailored assistance in the comfort of one's home, addressing personal care, meal preparation, and even medical needs. On the other hand, adult day centers provide social engagement and activities for the person with dementia, affording caregivers valuable time to attend to personal matters or simply rest.

Financing care is a practical aspect that cannot be overlooked. Many families face the challenge of managing the costs associated with professional care. Exploring insurance options, government assistance programs, and nonprofit resources can uncover avenues to subsidize these essential services.

The emotional journey of seeking and accepting help is punctuated with feelings of guilt and apprehension. It's natural to wrestle with these emotions; however, recognizing the benefits that respite and external help bring to both the caregiver and the recipient of care can ease these concerns. The act of allowing others to share in the caregiving responsibilities reinforces the notion that the journey is a collective effort.

Creating a care plan that includes regular intervals of respite can serve as a lifeline for caregivers. It's a structured approach that ensures the caregiver's health and emotional needs are not neglected. This plan can be as flexible as necessary, accommodating changes in the caregiver's or the loved one's condition.

Engaging with caregiver support groups, either in person or online, can provide a wealth of information and resources regarding respite care options and strategies for managing caregiver burnout. These communities offer not only practical advice but also emotional support, understanding, and the reassurance that you are not alone.

The involvement of family and friends plays a critical role in the caregiving ecosystem. Mobilizing this informal network to share the caregiving responsibilities can provide much-needed relief and support. It's also an opportunity for others to contribute positively to the loved one's care, fostering a sense of collective responsibility and community.

Documenting the care journey, including the tasks performed by caregivers and the roles external help fulfills, can provide clarity and structure. This documentation is particularly helpful when communicating needs to healthcare providers or coordinating care amongst multiple helpers.

Caregivers must remember the importance of maintaining their own health and happiness. Embracing respite and seeking external help are acts of self-care that enable caregivers to continue providing love and support with renewed energy and patience.

In the face of decision-making about the type and extent of external help to engage, it's vital to involve the person with dementia to the extent possible. Respect for their preferences and comfort levels should guide these decisions, ensuring that the care received is both effective and compassionate.

Tapping into local and national resources can uncover opportunities for support that caregivers might not be aware of. From funding assistance to free or low-cost respite care options, these resources are invaluable for caregivers looking to balance their roles and their own well-being.

Ultimately, embracing respite and external help is about finding balance in the caregiving journey. It's about acknowledging the limitations of what one person can do and recognizing the strength in asking for and accepting help. This balance allows caregivers to provide the best possible care while also living their own lives fully and with joy.

In closing, the journey of caregiving is one of love, sacrifice, and resilience. By embracing the need for respite and external help, caregivers can sustain their well-being and continue to provide compassionate care, ensuring a journey that is as rewarding as it is challenging.

Keeping Personal Connections Alive

Amid the taxing journey of providing care for a loved one with dementia, it's paramount to remember the importance of nurturing one's own relationships—those special bonds outside the caregiver-care recipient dynamic. Each interaction, each moment spent with a friend or family member, acts as a vital lifeline, a reminder of the world beyond the confines of care. This section aims to unfold methods and thoughts on maintaining these essential connections, ensuring the caregiver doesn't become isolated in their role.

Engaging in open dialogue with friends and family about the circumstances and challenges faced can establish a support network grounded in understanding and empathy. Sharing insights into daily realities not only informs but also invites loved ones to offer assistance, be it through offering respite, running errands, or simply lending an ear. Communication is the thread that ties these relationships together, preventing the fraying ends of isolation.

Scheduling regular outings with friends serves as a critical respite and a means to recharge one's emotional and mental batteries. Whether it's a simple coffee date, a walk in the park, or attending a local event, these moments away from caregiving responsibilities can rejuvenate the spirit and provide much-needed leisure and laughter. It's not a luxury but a necessity, marking reminders in one's calendar to prioritize these engagements.

Embracing technology to stay connected has never been more critical. With the advent of social media, video calls, and messaging apps, distance shrinks, allowing for frequent touchpoints with those who might not be physically near. A simple text message or a scheduled video call can bridge gaps, ensuring that relationships continue to flourish despite physical constraints.

Involving one's self in community activities or groups outside the caregiving sphere can lead to new friendships and connections, offering a fresh perspective and diversification of one's support network. Whether it's joining a book club, attending fitness classes, or volunteering, these activities allow for personal growth and social interaction, effectively counteracting feelings of isolation.

Maintaining hobbies or interests that are entirely separate from caregiving tasks can also serve as an important emotional outlet and means of self-expression. Whether it's painting, gardening, or playing an instrument, dedicating time to such activities fosters a sense of self and provides a break from the caregiver identity.

Setting boundaries is crucial to keeping personal connections alive. It's essential to communicate limits with the care recipient, if possible, and with other family members to ensure that personal time is respected and preserved. This might mean setting specific visiting hours or designating caregiving responsibilities to others during personal outings.

Seeking support from those who are navigating similar experiences, by joining a dementia caregiver support group, can lead to deep connections with people who truly understand the intricacies of caregiving. These groups often provide both emotional support and practical advice, offering a space where caregivers can share, listen, and connect on a profound level.

Being mindful of one's wellbeing and recognizing when to ask for help is fundamental. Friends and family are often willing to offer support but might not know how or when it is needed. Being open about specific needs—whether it's someone to talk to, assistance with caregiving tasks, or simply company—allows others to provide meaningful support.

Establishing a routine that includes social interaction is beneficial not just for the caregiver but also for the care recipient, when possible. Including the person with dementia in social activities can help maintain their social skills and provide them with stimulation, contributing positively to their well-being and allowing shared experiences amongst friends and family.

Dedication to personal relationships requires conviction; it's an active process of carving out time, engaging in meaningful conversations, and sometimes saying 'yes' to help. Balancing caregiving responsibilities with the need for personal connection can seem daunting, but it's through these efforts that caregivers can sustain their own well-being along this journey.

Utilizing respite care services, when available, can provide caregivers with the temporary relief needed to tend to personal relationships. Whether it's a professional service or a formal arrangement with friends/family, taking advantage of these opportunities is essential for maintaining balance.

Reflecting on the journey with loved ones, expressing gratitude for their presence and support, strengthens bonds. Gratitude, expressed through words or gestures, acknowledges the shared journey and honors the role each person plays in providing strength and comfort.

Finally, it's imperative to acknowledge that maintaining personal connections is a dynamic process; it evolves as the caregiving situation changes. Remaining flexible, open to change, and compassionate towards oneself is crucial in adapting to these shifts while keeping the essence of personal relationships intact.

In conclusion, the caregiver's journey is one of immense sacrifice and love, often placing the needs of another above one's own. Yet, in the midst of this profound commitment, it remains essential to nurture the personal connections that provide strength, joy, and respite. By actively engaging in the methods discussed, caregivers can safeguard their well-being and ensure that they, too, are supported and cherished as they support and cherish others.

Leaning on Support Networks and Professional Help

As one traverses the complex path of caregiving, the significance of support networks and professional guidance can't be overstressed. It's crucial to acknowledge that the journey isn't one to be embarked upon in isolation. Engaging with both local and online support groups provides a platform to share experiences, garner emotional support, and exchange practical advice with those in similar situations. Additionally, seeking professional help through counseling can offer a safe space to navigate one's feelings and develop coping strategies. Such resources not only serve as a lifeline in managing day-to-day stress but also empower caregivers to maintain their well-being. By leaning into these networks, caregivers find not only a semblance of relief but also a sense of community and understanding that bolsters resilience in the face of dementia's challenges.

Exploring Counseling and Support Group Options is an essential step for caregivers navigating the often turbulent waters of dementia care. The emotional and psychological toll it takes can sometimes be overwhelming, and finding a support structure through counseling and group sessions can provide much-needed relief and understanding. This exploration can be seen as an extension of one's commitment to providing the best care possible, not just for their loved one, but for themselves as well.

The journey starts with recognizing the signs that you might benefit from professional support or a community of others in similar situations. Feelings of isolation, frustration, sadness, and caregiver burnout are not uncommon. It's important to acknowledge these feelings and understand that seeking help is a sign of strength, not weakness.

One of the first options to consider is individual counseling. A professional therapist can offer a private space to express and work through the complex emotions tied to caregiving. They can provide coping strategies tailored to your specific situation, helping to navigate the unique challenges you face.

On the other hand, support groups offer a different kind of solace. These are gatherings of individuals who are all walking a path similar to yours. The power of shared experience can't be overstated—it creates a sense of community and understanding that is hard to find elsewhere. Here, you can share tips, provide emotional support for one another, and realize you're not alone in your journey.

Choosing between individual counseling and support groups—or opting for both—depends on your personal comfort level and what you feel will help you most. Some find the personal attention of counseling more beneficial, while others thrive in the communal aspect of support groups.

Finding a counselor or group that specializes in dementia care is crucial. These professionals and peers understand the nuances of the disease and can provide guidance that's both practical and empathetic. Your local health department, hospital, or Alzheimer's Association can be great places to start your search.

It's important to consider the logistics as well. Support groups, for example, meet at various times and locations. Some may find an online group more accessible, while others prefer the in-person connection. When it comes to counseling, check with your insurance provider to see what services are covered to make it as cost-effective as possible.

When you attend your first support group meeting or counseling session, it's normal to feel nervous or uncertain. Remember, every member started exactly where you are, and the group's purpose is to support one another. It's okay to simply listen until you're comfortable sharing.

Confidentiality is a cornerstone of both counseling and support groups. This understanding allows members to share openly and honestly, fostering a safe environment for healing and growth. It's this atmosphere of trust that facilitates the most profound connections and breakthroughs.

In addition to professional counseling and support groups, consider exploring structured caregiver training and educational programs. These can equip you with the skills needed to manage the practical aspects of caregiving while also addressing the emotional and psychological strains.

Throughout this journey, remember to be patient with yourself. Finding the right support system can take time, and what works for you might change as your caregiving situation evolves. The important thing is to stay open to the possibilities that support groups and counseling offer.

Document your experiences in caregiving and how these support options impact you. Keeping a journal can help you process your feelings and recognize your growth over time. It can also serve as a valuable tool for therapists or group members to better understand your challenges and victories.

Self-compassion is a critical component of the caregiving journey. Recognize that seeking support through counseling and groups is an act of self-care. It's essential to manage your own emotional and psychological health as you care for your loved one.

Lastly, encourage fellow caregivers to explore their options for support. As you find benefit in these resources, sharing your experiences can light the way for others who might be struggling in silence. Your journey could inspire others to seek the help they need, creating a ripple effect of support and understanding within the caregiving community.

Embracing counseling and support group options is not an admission of inadequacy; rather, it's a proactive step towards ensuring the well-being of both you and your loved one. By exploring these avenues, you pave the way for a more balanced, informed, and compassionate caregiving experience.

Connecting with Others through Online Platforms

In our journey as caregivers, the significance of maintaining and cultivating connections cannot be understated. In the digital age, online platforms have emerged as vital spaces for finding support, sharing experiences, and learning from others who walk a similar path. This chapter delves into how engaging with online communities can be a source of strength, solace, and practical advice for those caring for loved ones with dementia.

The advent of social media and specialized forums has indeed transformed the landscape of caregiver support. Websites dedicated to dementia care bring together individuals from all walks of life, offering a sense of belonging and understanding that can sometimes be elusive in our immediate environments. These platforms allow for the sharing of personal stories, which can illuminate the caregiving journey in profound ways, providing both comfort and insight.

Moreover, engaging in online support groups presents an opportunity to exchange practical advice on daily care strategies, behavioral management, and navigating healthcare systems. Often, these groups are moderated by professionals or experienced caregivers who can offer guidance backed by extensive knowledge and empathy. The interchange of tips and resources can be a lifeline for those facing new challenges in their caregiving roles.

It is, however, essential to approach online communities with discernment. The vast array of information available can sometimes overwhelm or lead to the dissemination of misinformation. It's advisable to verify shared advice with healthcare professionals and seek out reputable sources for information. This cautious approach ensures that the support and knowledge garnered from these platforms are both reliable and beneficial.

Email newsletters and blogs authored by caregiving experts and advocacy groups are another resource that can be accessed via online platforms. These written pieces often delve into topics ranging from emotional support to the latest research on dementia care, providing a wealth of knowledge that can be digested in one's own time.

The beauty of connecting through online platforms also lies in the diversity of experiences and perspectives it brings together. Caregivers can find solace in knowing they are not alone in facing the complexities and heartaches of dementia care. This collective wisdom fosters a unique camaraderie, reinforcing the notion that though the journey may be fraught with challenges, there is a community ready to uplift and support each other.

Participating in virtual events, such as webinars and live Q&A sessions with dementia care experts, is another way online platforms facilitate connection and learning. These events can provide up-to-date information and strategies for managing dementia care, along with the opportunity to engage directly with professionals and fellow caregivers.

Online platforms also offer the flexibility to engage in support networks on your terms and timetable. Whether it's contributing to a midnight discussion thread or browsing articles during a quiet morning, the 24/7 nature of the internet makes these resources accessible whenever they are needed most.

Privacy is another consideration that makes online interactions appealing. Many find comfort in the anonymity that online forums can provide, allowing for open and honest sharing of situations and feelings that might be difficult to express offline. This level of privacy can foster a more genuine exchange of advice and support.

The use of multimedia resources such as instructional videos and podcasts available on these platforms further enriches the caregiver's toolbox. Visual and auditory materials can offer a more engaging way to understand complex topics, from demonstrating caregiving techniques to providing relaxation exercises for stress relief.

Yet, for all the benefits that online platforms provide, it's crucial to remember the importance of offline connections as well. The human touch and presence of family, friends, and support groups hold an irreplaceable value. Online platforms should complement, rather than replace, the richness of direct human interaction.

Setting boundaries around the consumption of online content is also imperative. While these resources are invaluable, spending excessive time in digital spaces can inadvertently lead to information overload or exacerbate feelings of isolation. It's important to find a balance that enriches rather than overwhelms.

In conclusion, online platforms offer a vital lifeline for caregivers navigating the complex terrain of dementia care. They provide access to a global community of support, a wealth of information, and a source of comfort during the most challenging moments of the caregiving journey. By engaging with these digital spaces thoughtfully and responsibly, caregivers can harness the full potential of these resources to enhance both their own and their loved one's quality of life.

As we continue to explore the tender road of caregiving, let us embrace the opportunities for connection that online platforms provide. In doing so, we fortify ourselves against the isolation and challenges of dementia care, drawing strength from a community that understands, supports, and walks beside us every step of the way.

The embrace of technology in our caregiving journey reflects a modern approach to an age-old duty - attending to those we love with compassion, wisdom, and an open heart. It serves as a reminder that in the age of connectivity, no one needs to navigate the path of caregiving alone.

Chapter 6:
Managing Caregiver Stress with Compassion

Caregiving, by its very nature, is an act filled with compassion and love. It is a journey that requires one to tread tenderly, bearing a heart both strong and soft. Yet, this path is not without its thorns. The stress and emotional turmoil can, at times, seem overwhelming. In this chapter, we delve into strategies and practices designed to manage caregiver stress with the same compassion that inspires us to care for our loved ones.

First and foremost, it's crucial to acknowledge the legitimacy of your stress and emotional strain. It's not a sign of weakness, nor does it reflect a lack of devotion. Rather, it is a testament to your humanity and the depth of your care. By accepting this, you set the stage for a journey towards healing and balance.

Harnessing relaxation and stress reduction techniques can be a powerful antidote to the pressures of caregiving. Techniques such as deep breathing, meditation, and yoga are not just exercises for the body but balm for the soul. They offer moments of serenity in the midst of chaos, enabling you to return to your duties with a calmer, more centered spirit.

Deep breathing is perhaps the simplest yet most profound of these practices. It serves as an anchor, grounding you in moments of acute stress. By focusing on the rhythm of your breath, you can navigate through the stormiest of emotions, finding peace in the eye of the storm.

Meditation, too, invites you into a space of quiet reflection. It allows you to step back from your caregiver duties and touch base with your inner self. This practice can help illuminate the reasons behind your stress, making it easier to address them.

Yoga, on the other hand, nurtures both mind and body. Through its gentle stretches and poses, it releases the physical tension that stress often brings. Simultaneously, its focus on mindful movement encourages emotional release, healing the scars of caregiving stress.

Expressing emotions is another key strategy in managing stress. Keeping feelings bottled up only serves to increase internal pressure. Journaling offers a private, sacred space to lay bare your thoughts and emotions. It's a practice that can validate your feelings, providing clarity and relief.

Art, in its myriad forms, also provides a powerful outlet for emotional expression. Whether it's painting, drawing, or crafting, engaging in creative activities can help channel stress into something beautiful. Art transcends language, allowing you to communicate feelings that words cannot capture.

It's important to remember, however, that managing stress is not a solitary journey. Leaning on support networks, be they friends, family, or caregiver support groups, can provide much-needed relief. Sharing your experiences and hearing others' stories can foster a sense of community and understanding, reminding you that you are not alone.

Professional help, too, can be invaluable. Therapists and counselors specialize in helping people navigate through emotional turmoil. They can offer strategies tailored to your situation, helping you craft a personalized path towards well-being.

Lastly, remember to practice self-compassion. Be kind to yourself in moments of doubt and frustration. Recognize your efforts and forgive yourself for any perceived shortcomings. After all, caregiving is an act of love, and that includes loving yourself.

As we close this chapter, let us carry forward the message that managing stress is not merely about finding peace amidst chaos but about embracing our own humanity with compassion. For in doing so, we not only enhance our ability to care for our loved ones but also honor the depth of our own hearts.

In the journey of caregiving, let compassion be both your shield and your guiding light. With each deep breath, each moment of meditation or yoga, each word penned in a journal, and each stroke of the brush, let us nurture our spirits. For it is in caring for ourselves that we find the strength to care for others with unwavering love and patience.

Remember, in the complex tapestry of dementia care, managing stress with compassion is not just a chapter in a book but a chapter in your life. It's about weaving threads of resilience, kindness, and self-care into the very fabric of your caregiving journey. Let us tread this path with gentleness, both for our loved ones and ourselves, and keep alive the flame of hope and love that guides us through.

Harnessing Relaxation and Stress Reduction Techniques

In the labyrinth of challenges that come with caring for a loved one with dementia, it's crucial to remember the power of relaxation and stress reduction techniques for caregivers. The texture of our days can drastically change when we introduce practices such as deep breathing, meditation, and gentle yoga into our routine. These aren't just activities; they are bridges to a calmer state of being, where the burden on our shoulders feels lighter. Imagine the ripple effect on your well-being when you dedicate moments to simply breathe deeply, allowing each inhale to bring in peace and each exhale to release the weight of your worries. Meditation can become a refuge, a quiet room in your mind where you can rest and rejuvenate. Yoga, with its gentle stretches and mindful movements, can help release the tension that accumulates in your body from the physical demands of caregiving. It's about finding those small islands of tranquility in your day to cultivate resilience and sustain your compassion for the journey ahead. These techniques are not just beneficial; they're essential tools in maintaining both your physical and emotional health amidst the complexities of caregiving.

Incorporating Deep Breathing, Meditation, and Yoga into your caregiving routine could not only alleviate the stress you're under but also enhance the well-being of the loved one you're caring for. The journey through dementia is undoubtedly fraught with emotional and physical challenges, but embracing these time-honored practices can provide a much-needed sanctuary for both caregiver and care recipient.

In the hustle of managing the complex needs of a person with dementia, it's easy to overlook the powerful impact of deep breathing. This simple yet profound practice can reset your stress levels within minutes. By consciously taking slow, deep breaths, you signal your body to calm the fight or flight response, leading to a reduction in heart rate and a sense of peace. Guiding your loved one in this practice can be equally beneficial, as it promotes relaxation and can ease feelings of anxiety or agitation that often accompany cognitive decline.

Meditation, often perceived as a solitary exercise, can be a shared experience between you and your care recipient. The silence of the mind that meditation seeks to achieve may seem far-fetched when dealing with dementia's chaos. Yet, it's the concerted effort to quiet your thoughts and focus on the present that bears fruit. Initially, meditating for just a few minutes a day can introduce a sense of calm and connectedness amidst the turmoil. It helps in building patience and empathy, qualities essential in navigating the demanding role of a caregiver.

Yoga combines the benefits of deep breathing and meditation with physical movement, making it a holistic practice for stress relief and physical health. It's adaptable to all fitness levels and can be especially gentle for seniors. Incorporating yoga into your caregiving routine doesn't require rigorous sessions; instead, focus on simple poses and stretches that promote flexibility, balance, and muscle strength. Engaging in yoga together can become a productive, bonding activity that enhances mood and overall physical well-being.

The integration of these practices into daily life can begin with small steps. You might start with a five-minute deep breathing exercise each morning, gradually extending the time as it becomes a comfortable habit. Introducing meditation can follow, using guided sessions available through various apps or online resources that cater to all experience levels. As for yoga, many community centers and senior centers offer classes designed for older adults, which could be a wonderful outing for both of you.

Beyond the direct benefits to stress levels and physical health, these practices can profoundly affect the emotional connection between caregiver and care recipient. In moments of shared silence during meditation or mutual support in maintaining a yoga pose, there's an unspoken understanding and empathy that strengthens your bond. Dementia can often feel like a barrier that impedes emotional connection, but through these mindful practices, you're reminded of the enduring strength of your relationship.

It's also worth noting that deep breathing, meditation, and yoga can improve sleep quality — a common challenge in dementia care. Both you and your loved one might find it easier to relax and slip into a more restful sleep after engaging in these gentle, calming practices. This improvement in sleep can significantly impact your loved one's mood and behavior, potentially easing some of the daily caregiving challenges.

Moreover, these practices support emotional regulation, helping both the caregiver and the person with dementia to handle frustration, sadness, and anxiety more effectively. They provide tools for coping with the emotional rollercoaster that dementia often brings, offering a sense of control and resilience in the face of uncertainty.

Incorporating these practices requires patience and flexibility. It's important to approach them with an open mind and without expectations of perfection. The goal is not to achieve the ideal pose or a completely empty mind but to find moments of peace and connection amidst the day-to-day challenges of dementia care.

Additionally, the social aspect of participating in classes or groups for yoga or meditation can offer a reprieve from the isolation that often accompanies caregiving. These gatherings are opportunities to meet others on similar journeys, share experiences, and find community support. They serve as reminders that you're not alone in this journey, providing both social interaction and emotional uplift.

For caregivers who might feel hesitant or uncertain about how to begin, seeking out resources can be a helpful first step. Many books, websites, and local services provide guidance tailored to beginners. It's also helpful to communicate with your care recipient's healthcare provider before starting any new physical activities to ensure they're appropriate and safe.

Remember, the effectiveness of deep breathing, meditation, and yoga lies not just in their physical aspects but in their ability to nurture the mind and spirit as well. They are practices that honor the present moment, encourage acceptance, and foster a sense of inner peace — qualities invaluable to both caregivers and those receiving care.

In the end, the incorporation of these practices into your caregiving routine is an act of love and self-care. It's a recognition of the need for compassion, not only for the person you're caring for but for yourself as well. In the journey of dementia caregiving, where so much can feel out of control, these practices offer a sanctuary of calm and a pathway to resilience.

Embracing deep breathing, meditation, and yoga is more than just adding activities to your day; it's about creating space for peace, connection, and well-being in the midst of one of life's most challenging experiences. As you navigate the complex path of caring for a loved one with dementia, let these practices be your guideposts, illuminating the way with grace and strength.

Ultimately, the journey through dementia is a shared one, and incorporating these mindful practices can help in forging a path filled with moments of tranquility, understanding, and unconditional love. It is within these moments that the true essence of caregiving reveals itself, transforming both the caregiver and the care recipient in profound and unexpected ways.

Expressing Emotions through Journaling and Art

As we delve into the intricacies of caregiver stress and its myriad pressures, it's paramount we find solace in expressive outlets that not only alleviate the burden but also nurture the spirit. In the journey of caregiving, the emotional landscape can be as unpredictable as the condition we are battling against. Amidst the trials, journaling and art emerge not merely as activities, but as vessels for emotional expression and healing.

The act of journaling, often seen as a personal diary, is a profoundly therapeutic tool. It allows for the outpouring of thoughts and emotions in a raw, unfiltered manner. This exercise has the unique capability to bridge the gap between inner turmoil and a tangible form. For caregivers, setting aside time each day to jot down thoughts, feelings, and experiences can serve as a powerful release mechanism, lightening the emotional load and providing clarity amidst confusion.

It's not about eloquence or literary value when penning down your experiences; it's about authenticity. Let the words flow without concern for grammar or structure. It is in this freedom that many find relief. Additionally, journaling can become a record of the journey, reflecting both the struggles and the poignant moments of joy that light up this challenging path.

Parallel to journaling stands art, another expressive form that transcends verbal language. Art therapy has long been recognized for its healing properties, offering an expansive field where emotions, thoughts, and desires can be explored and expressed. For caregivers tethered to the demands of dementia care, art provides an escape, a momentary respite where the focus shifts from the care recipient to the caregiver's inner world.

Engaging in art doesn't require a background in fine arts or innate talent. The process itself is the therapy; whether it's painting, sketching, sculpting, or even crafting, the act of creating is what offers the emotional release. Art allows for a non-verbal conversation with oneself, uncovering and addressing feelings that might be too complex or painful to articulate in words.

Fusing both journaling and art into the caregiving routine can instill a sense of balance and personal fulfillment. These practices offer an exclusive space for caregivers to attend to their emotional needs, to acknowledge and process their feelings in a manner that champions self-expression and healing.

The integration of journaling and art into daily life need not be cumbersome or time-consuming. Starting with mere minutes a day can gradually unfold into a cherished part of your routine. Consider setting a specific time for these activities, creating a comforting ritual that you look forward to.

Moreover, it's essential to designate a private, tranquil space for these practices, where you can immerse in the process without interruptions. This personal sanctuary becomes a symbol of self-care, a physical manifestation of the importance of tending to one's emotional health amidst the demands of caregiving.

If uncertainty or hesitation arises when staring at a blank page or canvas, remember that there is no right or wrong way to express oneself. The objective is not to create a masterpiece but to find an outlet for emotions, to discover solace and understanding through the act of creation.

Sharing your art or journal entries can also be a potent way to connect with others, especially those in similar situations. Caregiver support groups, both in person and online, often welcome such expressions, understanding the therapeutic value and offering a platform for shared experiences and mutual understanding.

In times of extreme strain, when emotions are too overwhelming to articulate or transform into art, these expressive forms can still serve you. Simply being present with your journal or art supplies, acknowledging your need for this time, can be a form of self-care and acknowledgment of your feelings.

Embedding expressive practices like journaling and art into the fabric of your life doesn't just help manage stress; it enriches your personal journey. It transforms caregiving from a task solely focused on the physical and cognitive decline of a loved one, to an experience that encompasses growth, reflection, and emotional resilience for the caregiver.

As the journey with dementia unfolds, it becomes clear that caring for a loved one also means caring for oneself. Embracing journaling and art as parts of your caregiving strategy empowers you to face the challenges with a stronger, more resilient spirit.

Recognize that in moments of doubt or loneliness, your journal or canvas can be a silent yet profound companion, holding space for your emotions and thoughts. They offer solace, understanding, and sometimes, the clarity needed to navigate the complex path of caregiving.

Finally, let us remember that in expressing ourselves through journaling and art, we are not retreating from our duties but equipping ourselves with strength. We are acknowledging that to provide the best care to our loved ones, we must first tend to our emotional well-being. Through these acts of self-expression, we find the courage to continue, to face each day with hope and a renewed sense of purpose.

Chapter 7:
Nurturing Connections Throughout Dementia's Journey

The progression of dementia presents a series of challenges, both for the person experiencing the condition and those around them. However, amidst the trials, fostering a deep and meaningful connection becomes profoundly significant. It is through the nurturing of these connections that both caregivers and those in their care can find solace, companionship, and joy.

One of the most effective ways to maintain a connection is through engaging in sensory activities. These can include listening to music, sharing a meal, or taking part in gentle physical activity together. Such experiences can stir memories and emotions, providing common ground for conversation and interaction.

Reminiscence, or sharing memories from the past, serves as another powerful tool in strengthening bonds. Discussing familiar stories, looking at old photographs, or visiting memorable places can evoke feelings of comfort and happiness, for both the caregiver and the person with dementia.

It's equally important to embrace moments of joy and celebration, no matter how small. Recognizing and appreciating the positive experiences that occur despite the disease can help dispel the clouds of despair. Celebrating milestones, enjoying a laugh, or simply savoring a peaceful moment together can uplift everyone's spirits.

Yet, cultivating these connections goes beyond engaging in activities; it requires patience, understanding, and empathy. It means entering their world without judgement, embracing their reality, and offering support in a manner that respects their dignity and individuality.

Understanding non-verbal cues becomes crucial in this context. As dementia progresses, verbal communication may diminish, making it imperative for caregivers to become attuned to expressions, gestures, and even silence. These non-verbal signals can convey a wealth of feelings and needs, allowing for continued interaction and bonding.

Adapting to the changing dynamics of the relationship is another vital aspect. Recognizing the evolving needs of the person with dementia and adjusting your approach accordingly can aid in sustaining a nurturing connection. This might mean simplifying activities, offering more direct assistance, or finding new ways to communicate love and care.

Maintaining a sense of humor can also be a powerful ally. Laughter not only relieves stress but can also help bridge gaps created by cognitive decline. It's a way to share moments of light-heartedness, forging connections through joy rather than sorrow.

Encouraging social interaction, as much as possible, serves to enrich the lives of those with dementia. Interacting with others, whether family, friends, or even pets, can stimulate feelings of belonging and joy. Caregivers can facilitate these interactions by arranging small gatherings or simply integrating social activities into daily routines.

It's also beneficial to establish a community of support that includes other caregivers and professionals. Sharing experiences, challenges, and successes with those who understand can provide emotional buoyancy and insightful strategies for nurturing connections.

Integrating technology can offer additional avenues for engagement. Utilizing video calls, digital photo albums, or apps designed for dementia care can enhance communication and provide enjoyable shared experiences.

Remaining flexible and open to change is paramount. As dementia progresses, the abilities and interests of the person may shift. Recognizing and adapting to these changes can foster an environment where connections continue to thrive despite new challenges.

Finally, it's essential to look after oneself. A caregiver's ability to nurture connections largely depends on their own well-being. Self-care isn't just beneficial for the caregiver; it's crucial for maintaining the capacity to provide compassionate and effective care.

In conclusion, nurturing connections throughout dementia's journey is a dynamic and fluid process. It requires creativity, patience, and resilience. Yet, the rewards of maintaining these bonds are immeasurable, offering glimpses of joy, shared laughter, and moments of profound connection that illuminate the path for both the caregiver and the person with dementia.

As we draw this chapter to a close, let us carry forward the understanding that amidst the inevitable challenges of dementia, the capacity for human connection remains an indomitable force. It's within these connections that we find the strength to continue, the grace to accept each day, and the joy in moments that become memories cherished forever.

Fostering Emotional Bonding and Positive Encounters

In the heart of the journey with dementia, amidst the complexities and the shifting landscapes of care, lies the golden thread of fostering emotional bonding and positive encounters. It's about paving a path of understanding and empathy, recognizing that each moment holds the potential for connection, regardless of the stage or severity of dementia. This endeavor calls for a blend of creativity and patience, as one navigates the terrain of memory loss and cognitive decline. Engaging in activities that ignite the senses and evoke memories can act as a bridge between worlds, enabling caregivers and their loved ones to meet in a space of shared experiences. Whether it's through the gentle touch of a hand, the shared laughter over a familiar song, or the warmth of sitting together in silence, these moments of connection are invaluable. They remind us that at the heart of care is the nurturing of the human spirit, fostering encounters that transcend the spoken word and nurturing a bond that endures the ravages of time.

Engaging through Sensory Activities and Reminiscence is a vital approach for maintaining connections and enhancing the quality of life for those living with dementia. Over time, memories may become elusive, and the world a bit more confusing, but the senses remain powerful gateways to the past and present. Engaging a person with dementia through sensory activities and reminiscence can awaken emotions, memories, and even moments of clarity that seemed beyond reach.

The power of touch cannot be underestimated, particularly in the later stages of dementia. A simple act of holding hands, a gentle massage of the shoulders, or brushing their hair can provide comfort and a sense of security. These tactile experiences can also stimulate memories and emotions, providing a bridge to moments of personal significance. Remember, the skin is the largest sensory organ and remains responsive long after other senses have diminished.

Aromas have a unique ability to transport us back in time. Imagine the scent of a favorite meal cooking, a perfume worn in younger years, or the smell of fresh-cut grass. These fragrances can evoke vivid memories, often linked to emotions and experiences. For someone with dementia, smelling lavender might recall memories of gardening, while the scent of vanilla could bring back the warmth of holiday baking. Such scent-based activities can offer a reassuring sense of familiarity.

The introduction of familiar music and sounds is another enriching sensory activity. Playing songs from their youth, favorite hymns, or the sound of rain and nature can soothe, stimulate, and sometimes unlock the doors to lost memories. It's not uncommon for individuals with dementia to remember and sing along to songs from their past, even when verbal communication has become challenging. Music can also encourage movement, such as clapping, dancing, or tapping a foot, providing both a physical and emotional outlet.

Taste and food experiences play a significant role in our lives and can be a source of pleasure for someone with dementia. Preparing and sharing a meal that was a past favorite can be a powerful act of reminiscence. The act of cooking together, when possible, or simply enjoying a beloved dish can trigger memories of family gatherings, celebrations, and traditions. Additionally, involving individuals in simple food preparation tasks can help to engage their senses and foster feelings of accomplishment.

Visual cues are immensely helpful in sparking memories and encouraging conversation. Creating a reminiscence box or a scrapbook filled with photographs, mementos, and keepsakes from different times in their life offers a tangible link to their past. Flipping through old photos, touching familiar objects, or even watching videos from special occasions can prompt stories and recollections, facilitating connection and communication.

Gardening or interacting with nature engages multiple senses simultaneously – the feel of the soil, the sight of the blooming flowers, the smell of fresh herbs. These activities not only provide sensory stimulation but also a sense of calm and purpose. Being outdoors, when feasible, allows for natural light exposure, which can help regulate sleep patterns and improve overall well-being.

Animal interactions have been shown to have a calming effect on individuals with dementia. Whether it's a therapy animal visit or spending time with a family pet, the presence of animals can encourage tactile engagement, movement, and emotional expression. The unconditional love of an animal can offer comfort, reduce stress, and increase social interaction.

Engaging individuals with dementia through art and crafting activities can offer a non-verbal way to express themselves. Painting, coloring, or working with clay can stimulate the brain, evoke emotions, and offer a sense of accomplishment. Even if the individual struggles with cognitive tasks, the act of creating can provide an outlet for expression and foster a connection to the present moment.

Storytelling and shared reading are activities that can resonate deeply. Reading aloud from a favorite book or telling stories from the past can not only be comforting but also stimulate memories and conversation. Encouraging the person with dementia to tell their story can help maintain their sense of identity and provide insight into their experiences and emotions.

Simple everyday activities, such as folding laundry or organizing a drawer, can offer sensory stimulation and a sense of normalcy. These tasks can provide an opportunity for engagement, success, and the pleasant sensations associated with handling different textures.

Creating a sensory garden or space within the home can offer accessible and ongoing sensory stimulation. Incorporating plants, herbs, textured paths, and tranquil sounds can create a soothing environment that stimulates the senses and provides a refuge from overstimulation.

Light physical activities, adapted to the individual's abilities, such as walking, stretching, or simple seated exercises, can provide sensory feedback through movement. These activities help to maintain mobility, improve mood, and encourage a connection to the body and the environment.

Participating in community or social events that cater to individuals with dementia can offer a sense of belonging and new sensory experiences in a supportive setting. Whether it's music performances, art exhibitions, or nature walks, these outings can stimulate engagement and provide enjoyable experiences for both the individual and their caregiver.

In conclusion, engaging individuals with dementia through sensory activities and reminiscence is not just about triggering memories but about fostering connection, enhancing well-being, and enriching the daily life experience. Each person will respond differently to sensory engagement, so observing their reactions and adapting activities to their preferences and abilities is crucial. The goal is to create moments of joy, comfort, and a sense of meaning, contributing to a higher quality of life throughout their journey with dementia.

Embracing Moments of Joy and Celebration

In the intricate tapestry of caring for a loved one with dementia, it's crucial to remember the threads of joy that bind us together, even in the midst of challenges. Embracing moments of joy and celebration isn't just about marking birthdays or anniversaries; it's about recognizing and savoring the small victories and spontaneous smiles that occur daily. Whether it's the warmth of a shared laugh, the brief flicker of recognition in their eyes, or the pleasure found in listening to a favorite song together, these moments are rays of sunshine in the fog of dementia. To nurture connections throughout dementia's journey, actively seek out and create opportunities for positive experiences.

Celebrate the good days, no matter how rare they may seem, and allow those memories to fuel your resilience. This approach doesn't ignore the reality of the situation but adds a layer of richness to the caregiving experience that can help sustain both you and your loved one through this journey.

Recognizing and Savoring Positive Experiences in the context of dementia care can often feel like looking for a needle in a haystack. The terrain of caregiving is fraught with challenges and moments of despair. However, amidst this turbulent journey, there lie hidden pockets of joy, tenderness, and connection that can provide a much-needed respite for both the caregiver and the person with dementia. Recognizing and celebrating these moments is not just beneficial; it's essential for maintaining emotional health and resilience.

Caring for a loved one with dementia means adapting to a new rhythm of life, one that may often feel unpredictable. Yet, it's within this unpredictability that we can find surprising moments of clarity and connection. It may come in the form of a shared laugh, a moment of unexpected lucidity, or a tender gesture. These instances, fleeting as they may be, are significant. They remind us that the essence of the person we love is still present. Recognizing these moments requires a shift in focus, from dwelling on what has been lost to celebrating what remains.

The simple act of savoring involves being fully present and absorbing the joy in the moment. It's about letting go of the past and the future, if only for a second, and allowing oneself to be enveloped in the present experience. This might seem a monumental task amidst the duties and concerns of caregiving, but it's precisely these moments that can replenish our emotional reserves and strengthen our resilience.

To begin, it helps to consciously look for positive experiences each day. This might mean noticing the warmth in your loved one's eyes, the grip of their hand, or the inflection in their voice that reminds you of happier times. Pay attention to these details, as they are the building blocks of positive experiences that can light up the caregiving journey.

Creating opportunities for these experiences is equally important. This can involve engaging in activities that your loved one enjoys and is able to participate in, despite their cognitive decline. Music, for instance, has a unique way of reaching through the fog of dementia, invoking memories, and eliciting positive emotions. Similarly, looking through old photos, enjoying a favorite meal together, or spending time in nature can stimulate senses and evoke happiness.

Once you've recognized a positive moment, the next step is to savor it. Share your joy with your loved one, even if their understanding seems limited. Your emotional expression can be contagious, and it can create an atmosphere of warmth and love. Describe what you're feeling, smile, laugh, and make eye contact. These are all powerful ways of connecting and sharing the joy.

Journaling about these experiences can also enrich the savoring process. Writing down the details of these moments allows you to relive them and reflect on the joy they brought you. This practice can be a source of comfort on difficult days, reminding you of the good times amidst the challenges.

Encouraging family and friends to share in these positive experiences can amplify their impact. Sharing stories of joyful moments can foster a sense of community and support, reminding you that you're not alone on this journey. Plus, hearing others' perspectives on these experiences can deepen your appreciation and understanding of their significance.

It's also vital to celebrate small victories. Perhaps your loved one remembered a family member's name or managed to complete a simple task. These achievements, no matter how small, are monumental in the context of dementia. Acknowledging and celebrating them reinforces a sense of accomplishment and value for both you and your loved one.

Adopting a habit of gratitude can further deepen the ability to recognize and savor positive experiences. Each day, try to identify something you're grateful for, related to your caregiving journey. It could be the support of a friend, a resource that proved helpful, or simply a peaceful moment shared in silence. Gratitude shifts your focus from what is lacking to the abundance that exists, even in the midst of hardship.

While it's essential to recognize and savor positive experiences, it's also important to acknowledge that not every day will bring visible reasons to celebrate. There will be days filled with frustration, sadness, and fatigue. On these days, it's critical to practice self-compassion and remind yourself that it's okay to feel overwhelmed. Caring for someone with dementia is an immense task, and it's only natural to experience a wide range of emotions.

In these moments of despair, it can be helpful to return to your journal or to reach out to a support network. Sharing your feelings, whether they're of joy or sorrow, can lighten your emotional load. It's important to remember that experiencing joy does not negate the challenges of caregiving; rather, it coexists with them, providing balance and perspective.

The journey of dementia caregiving is undoubtedly marked by loss and change, but it's also punctuated with instances of love, joy, and connection. Recognizing and savoring these positive experiences can illuminate the path forward, providing moments of relief and reminders of the enduring bond between caregiver and loved one.

In conclusion, amidst the thorns of dementia care, there bloom roses of shared humanity and moments of connection. By recognizing and savoring these positive experiences, caregivers can find strength, hope, and moments of joy on a challenging journey. While the path may be uneven, the journey is rich with moments that remind us of the resilience of the human spirit and the enduring power of love.

Chapter 8:
Embracing the Tender Road

The journey of caring for someone with dementia is undeniably challenging, yet it's woven with moments of profound tenderness and beauty. As we draw near the conclusion of this guide, it's essential to pause and reflect on the resilient tapestry of care, love, and unyielding strength that each caregiver weaves every day. The road, as we have seen, is fraught with obstacles, but it's also lined with opportunities for growth, bonding, and understanding.

In the chapters that preceded, we ventured through the various landscapes that define the care journey - understanding the medical and emotional facets of dementia, adjusting the living environment for safety and comfort, and prioritizing self-care to sustain the caregiver's well-being. Yet, as we near the end, the focus shifts to a broader, more holistic view of this journey, embracing it not just as a challenge but as a profound, life-altering expedition.

This tender road compels us to recognize our own strengths and vulnerabilities. It teaches us that amidst the erosion of memory and cognition, the essence of the person we care for remains. Their joys, fears, and the core of their identity persist, demanding our respect, compassion, and, above all, our love.

It's a road that asks us to be present, to show up not just with solutions but with our hearts open, ready to connect in whatever ways possible. This may mean rediscovering the simple pleasures of tactile sensations, music, and shared smiles. It's about finding joy in the moment, however fleeting it may be.

Embracing the tender road means accepting that our efforts might not be remembered, but they will be felt. It acknowledges that while we cannot alter the course of the disease, we can influence the quality of the journey, ensuring it is laden with dignity, warmth, and respect.

It's also on this path that we learn the value of community and support. Reaching out for help, leaning on the strength of others, and sharing our experiences can illuminate our journey, making the road less daunting. Support networks, both in-person and online, remind us that we're not alone in our struggles.

Importantly, this journey reshapes our understanding of success. In a realm where conventional achievements are overshadowed by loss and decline, success is redefined as moments of connection, tranquillity, and mutual respect. It's found in the quiet appreciation of being together, in the strength we muster each day, and in the care we provide.

This road also teaches us about the ephemeral nature of life itself, reminding us to cherish each moment, to find beauty in the now, and to love fiercely and without reservation. It prompts us to forgive quickly, to let go of the trivial, and to hold tightly to what truly matters.

As caregivers, we're not just guardians of physical health but keepers of spirits. Our role is to nurture the flame of who our loved ones once were and still are, ensuring that the warmth of their essence is not extinguished by the fog of dementia.

Embracing the tender road is, ultimately, a journey of love. It's a testament to the human spirit's capacity for compassion, resilience, and boundless love. It's a road paved with heartache, yes, but also with immeasurable beauty and grace.

In closing, I invite you to view this journey not as a burden but as one of life's most profound honors. To care for someone on this path is to witness the spectrum of human existence, to experience love in its most unvarnished form. It may be a road marked by loss, but it is also a path rich with the essence of what it means to truly live and love.

So, let's walk this tender road together, embracing each challenge as an opportunity to grow, to connect, and to honor the deep, indelible bonds of love that define our shared humanity. May this guide serve as a beacon, illuminating your path with hope, strength, and compassion.

Remember, in the shadow of dementia, love is the light that endures. It's our guide on this tender road, leading us through the darkness with grace, illuminating our journey with moments of profound beauty and connection. It's love that ultimately triumphs, love that endures, and love that transforms this challenging journey into a tender, unforgettable odyssey of the heart.

In contemplating the road we've traveled and the path that lies ahead, let us hold fast to love. For it is in loving and being loved that we find the true essence of the human spirit. This, perhaps, is the greatest lesson of all: in the end, love is what matters most on this tender road we travel together.

Appendix:
Resources for Caregivers

In the journey of caregiving, having a trusted compendium of resources can dramatically ease the weight upon your shoulders. The following collection has been curated to guide you, the caregiver, through the labyrinth of tasks and emotions that accompany the care of a loved one with dementia.

Local and National Support Networks

Navigating the choppy waters of dementia caregiving necessitates a sturdy network of support. Below, you'll find a lighthouse - organizations dedicated to providing guidance, support, and companionship to those treading this tender road:

- **The Alzheimer's Association** (*alz.org*) – Offers a goldmine of information on Alzheimer's and other dementias, alongside a 24/7 helpline, support groups, and educational workshops.

- **The Family Caregiver Alliance** (*caregiver.org*) – Focuses on the needs of families and friends providing long-term care at home, offering educational resources, state-by-state help, and support groups.

- **The National Institute on Aging** (*nia.nih.gov*) – Provides comprehensive information on health and aging, with a rich section devoted to Alzheimer's and dementia care.

- **AARP's Caregiving Resource Center** (*aarp.org/caregiving*) – Offers advice on legal issues, health, and family dynamics along with interactive tools to customize your caregiving plan.

Essential Tools and Checklists for Dementia Care

Equip yourself with the right tools to manage the multifaceted responsibilities of caregiving efficiently. Here's a set of essential tools and checklists tailored to assist you in providing compassionate care:

1. **Daily Care Plan:** A comprehensive tool that helps maintain a consistent routine, ensuring all physical, emotional, and medical needs of your loved one are met.

2. **Safety Checklist:** A thorough assessment to secure your home and create a safe environment, minimizing the risk of wandering and accidents.

3. **Medication Management System:** Simplify the complex task of medication management to avoid missed doses and drug interactions, ensuring your loved one's health and wellbeing.

4. **Legal and Financial Planning Kit:** Early planning eases the strain on caregivers. This kit helps you organize documents and understand options for managing your loved one's affairs.

5. **Self-Care Schedule for Caregivers:** Equally important is a tool for scheduling self-care activities, highlighting the importance of caregiver health to sustain the journey ahead.

Remember, you're not alone on this journey. These resources are here to support and guide you through the challenges of caregiving. Leveraging them can help you find some solace and strength, allowing you to provide the best possible care to your loved one while also taking care of yourself.

Local and National Support Networks

The journey of caregiving is strewn with both joys and challenges, its path often winding and unexpected. Amidst the complexities of caring for a loved one with dementia, finding a robust support network can be akin to discovering a lighthouse in a storm. This chapter aims to illuminate the local and national support networks that stand ready to assist caregivers in their noble yet demanding role.

At the heart of local support networks are the community centers and healthcare facilities that often host groups for caregivers. These groups provide a haven where individuals can share their experiences, challenges, and triumphs with those who truly understand. Engaging with your local Alzheimer's Association chapter or similar organizations can offer opportunities to connect with these vital resources.

National support networks, meanwhile, extend their reach across the country, offering guidance, information, and advocacy. Organizations such as the Alzheimer's Association and the National Institute on Aging are pillars in the caregiver support landscape, providing up-to-date research, educational materials, and policy advocacy. Their websites and helplines serve as critical lifelines, offering support at both general and specialized levels.

One cannot overlook the role of online platforms in today's interconnected world. Forums, social media groups, and websites dedicated to dementia care have flourished, allowing caregivers to find support and camaraderie without geographic constraints. These online communities are not only platforms for sharing practical advice but also spaces for emotional support and understanding.

In recognizing the diverse needs of caregivers, many support networks also offer resources tailored to specific types of dementia, cultural backgrounds, and languages. This inclusive approach ensures that every caregiver can access support that resonates with their unique situation and caregiving journey.

Furthermore, for those who may struggle with transport or time constraints, virtual support groups present an invaluable alternative. These groups meet via video calls, making support accessible right from the comfort of one's home. This flexibility helps to ensure that all caregivers can find a sense of community and support, regardless of their circumstances.

Respite care services, though not a 'network' in the traditional sense, play a crucial role in supporting caregivers. Local health services and national organizations often provide directories to respite care options, giving caregivers the much-needed opportunity to rest and recharge while knowing their loved ones are in safe hands.

Educational workshops and seminars, frequently offered by these support networks, arm caregivers with knowledge about dementia care strategies, legal considerations, and health care planning. This education empowers caregivers, reducing the uncertainties that can accompany dementia care.

Legal and financial advice is another critical component of support networks. Given the complex nature of legal and financial planning in dementia care, many organizations offer guidance to help caregivers navigate these daunting territories. This can include information on power of attorney, guardianship, and accessing benefits.

Advocacy efforts are a significant focus for national support organizations, striving for greater public awareness and improved care policies. Caregivers are often encouraged to get involved in advocacy work, lending their voices to shape better futures for those affected by dementia.

In embracing the support offered by these networks, caregivers can also find strength in shared advocacy, contributing to a greater understanding and better care standards for dementia nationwide.

It's essential for caregivers to remember that they're not alone in their journey. By reaching out to local and national support networks, caregivers can find solace in shared experiences, gain new insights into the complexities of care, and find respite in knowing that a community of support surrounds them.

To effectively navigate these networks, caregivers are encouraged to keep an updated list of contacts for local and national support options. Regularly visiting their websites and participating in community events can help caregivers stay informed about new resources and support opportunities.

Lastly, building a personal network of support among family, friends, and fellow caregivers can complement the formal support provided by organizations. This network of personal connections forms the bedrock of emotional support, enabling caregivers to share not just the burden of care but also the moments of joy and fulfillment that come with it.

In closing, the role of local and national support networks in the lives of caregivers cannot be overstated. By tapping into these resources, caregivers can find the guidance, support, and community necessary to navigate the caregiving journey with resilience and grace. As we continue to explore the resources available to caregivers, it becomes ever more apparent that while the journey may be arduous, no one needs to travel it alone.

Essential Tools and Checklists for Dementia Care

Embarking on the journey of caregiving for a loved one with dementia is a path wrought with challenges, uncertainties, and occasional surprises. In such a scenario, being equipped with the right tools and checklists doesn't just offer a semblance of control but becomes a vital strategy for managing day-to-day tasks efficiently. This section delves into some indispensable resources that every caregiver should have in their arsenal to ensure the well-being of both themselves and their care recipients.

First and foremost, a detailed care plan document is an essential tool that cannot be overlooked. Such a document outlines the care recipient's medical conditions, medication schedules, dietary restrictions, and preferences. It serves as a guide for not just the primary caregiver but for any family member or professional stepping into help. A well-drafted care plan ensures continuity of care and minimizes misunderstandings or errors in the person's care regimen.

Daily task checklists are equally important and offer a structured approach to caregiving. These lists can include medication timings, meal plans, appointment schedules, and personal hygiene routines. By breaking down the day into manageable tasks, caregivers can ensure that all necessary activities are completed and can also track changes in the care recipient's needs or abilities over time.

Another vital aspect of dementia care involves safety measures. A safety checklist for the home can significantly reduce the risk of accidents or wandering incidents. This might include securing locks on windows and doors, installing night lights to prevent falls, and removing tripping hazards. Through regular review and adherence to a comprehensive safety checklist, caregivers can create a secure environment that supports the independence of the person with dementia as much as possible.

Mental stimulation activities are key in slowing down cognitive decline, and having a checklist of such activities can be beneficial. This could comprise puzzles, memory games, music sessions, or simple gardening projects. Tailoring activities to align with the individual's interests and abilities not only provides a sense of joy and accomplishment but also fosters emotional connection and engagement.

Moreover, nutritional care cannot be understated. A nutrition checklist ensures that meals are balanced, dietary restrictions are observed, and proper hydration is maintained. Nutritional neglect can lead to a plethora of health issues, making it crucial for caregivers to plan and monitor meal intake meticulously.

Another indispensable tool in the caregiver's toolkit is a medical appointment tracker. Keeping track of doctor's appointments, therapy sessions, and any other professional consultations is crucial for managing the health of someone with dementia effectively. This tracker can also be used to jot down questions or concerns to address during these visits, ensuring that all aspects of the person's health are covered.

Emergency contacts list and medical information sheet are crucial documents that should be easily accessible. In case of an emergency, having this information at hand can save valuable time and ensure that accurate information is shared with healthcare professionals.

Evaluating caregiver support needs is equally important. Caregivers should maintain a checklist to assess their own well-being, identify signs of burnout, and recognize when it's time to seek help. This could include reminders to schedule time for self-care activities or to reach out to support networks when overwhelmed.

Technology can also play a significant role in dementia care. Numerous apps and devices are designed to aid in medication management, appointment reminders, and even tracking the location of a person with dementia should they wander. Familiarizing oneself with technological aids that can make the caregiving process more seamless is highly beneficial.

Lastly, legal and financial documents checklist ensures that all critical paperwork is in order. This includes wills, powers of attorney, advanced healthcare directives, and insurance documents. Having these documents organized and updated can alleviate potential future stressors for the family.

In conclusion, being armed with these tools and checklists allows caregivers to navigate the complexities of dementia care with greater confidence and efficiency. It helps in creating a structured and safe environment for the person with dementia, while also safeguarding the mental and physical well-being of the caregiver. Remember, caregiving is not a journey to be embarked upon alone; these tools, combined with the support of family, friends, and professionals, can make a significant difference in the quality of care provided.

While the task of caregiving for someone with dementia can seem daunting, it's important to remember that resources are available to help. By utilizing these essential tools and checklists, you're not just performing tasks; you're enhancing the quality of life for your loved one and yourself. The road may be long and tender, but with the right preparation and support, moments of joy and connection remain within reach.

Thus, let these tools serve as your compass and guide on this caregiving journey. Embrace the resources at your disposal, adjust and adapt as necessary, and take comfort in knowing you're providing compassionate and comprehensive care to your loved one. Together, with patience and perseverance, you can navigate the challenges of dementia care and foster moments of joy and fulfillment amidst the journey.

www.ingramcontent.com/pod-product-compliance
Lightning Source LLC
Chambersburg PA
CBHW030344290526
45785CB00004B/1586